T0204154

# Forensic Anthropology and the United States Judicial System

# Published and forthcoming titles in the Forensic Science in Focus Series

## Published

*The Global Practice of Forensic Science*
Douglas H. Ubelaker (Editor)

*Forensic Chemistry: Fundamentals and Applications*
Jay A. Siegel (Editor)

*Forensic Microbiology*
David O. Carter, Jeffrey K. Tomberlin, M. Eric Benbow, and Jessica L. Metcalf (Editors)

*Forensic Anthropology: Theoretical Framework and Scientific Basis*
Clifford Boyd and Donna Boyd (Editors)

*The Future of Forensic Science*
Daniel A. Martell (Editor)

*Forensic Anthropology and the United States Judicial System*
Laura C. Fulginiti, Kristen Hartnett-McCann, and Alison Galloway (Editors)

## Forthcoming

*Forensic Science and Humanitarian Action: Interacting with the Dead and the Living*
Roberto C. Parra, Sara C. Zapico, and Douglas H. Ubelaker (Editors)

*Humanitarian Forensics and Human Identification*
Paul Emanovsky and Shuala M. Drawdy (Editors)

# Forensic Anthropology and the United States Judicial System

EDITED BY

## Laura C. Fulginiti

Maricopa County Office of the Medical Examiner
Arizona, USA

## Kristen Hartnett-McCann

State of Connecticut Office of the Chief Medical Examiner
Connecticut, USA

## Alison Galloway

University of California, Santa Cruz
USA

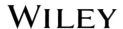

The right of Laura C. Fulginiti, Kristen Hartnett-McCann, and Alison Galloway to be identified as the authors of the editorial material in this work asserted in accordance with law.

*Registered Offices*
John Wiley & Sons, Inc., 111 River Street, Hoboken, NJ 07030, USA
9600 Garsington Road, Oxford, OX4 2DQ, UK

*Editorial Office*
John Wiley & Sons Ltd, The Atrium, Southern Gate, Chichester, West Sussex, PO19 8SQ, UK

For details of our global editorial offices, customer services, and more information about Wiley products visit us at www.wiley.com.

Wiley also publishes its books in a variety of electronic formats and by print-on-demand. Some content that appears in standard print versions of this book may not be available in other formats.

*Library of Congress Cataloging-in-Publication Data*

Names: Fulginiti, Laura C., editor. | Hartnett-McCann, Kristen, editor. |
    Galloway, Alison, 1953- editor.
Title: Forensic anthropology and the United States judicial system / [edited
    by] Laura C. Fulginiti, Kristen Hartnett-McCann, Alison Galloway.
Description: First edition. | Hoboken, NJ : Wiley, 2019. | Series: Forensic
    science in focus | Includes bibliographical references and index. |
    Identifiers: LCCN 2019015125 (print) | LCCN 2019015571 (ebook) | ISBN
    9781119470038 (Adobe PDF) | ISBN 9781119469971 (ePub) | ISBN 9781119470052
    (hardback)
Subjects: | MESH: Forensic Anthropology–methods | Expert Testimony–methods
    | United States
Classification: LCC GN69.8 (ebook) | LCC GN69.8 (print) | NLM W 750 | DDC
    614/.17–dc23
LC record available at https://lccn.loc.gov/2019015125

Cover Design: Wiley
Cover Image: Courtesy of Gary Hodges, Litigation Graphics Specialist

Set in size of 10.5/13.5pt and MeridienLTStd by SPi Global, Chennai, India
Printed and bound in Singapore by Markono Print Media Pte Ltd

10  9  8  7  6  5  4  3  2  1

*This volume is dedicated to Dr. Walter Hudson Birkby*

# Contents

# Notes on contributors

**Eric J. Bartelink, PhD, D-ABFA,** has taught for 13 years at California State University, Chico, where he is currently a full professor and director of the Human Identification Laboratory. His research interests focus on the bioarchaeology of Native California, dietary reconstruction using stable isotope analysis and applications within forensic anthropology. He is a coauthor of *Essentials of Physical Anthropology, Introduction to Physical Anthropology,* and *Forensic Anthropology: Current Methods and Practice* and has authored and coauthored numerous articles in scientific journals.

**Jonathan D. Bethard, PhD, D-ABFA**, is currently an Assistant Professor in the Department of Anthropology at the University of South Florida. He received his PhD in Anthropology from the University of Tennessee-Knoxville. Dr. Bethard specializes in forensic anthropology and bioarchaeology and has worked as a consultant in forensic anthropology for the International Criminal Investigative Training Assistance Program (ICITAP) in Colombia and Algeria as well the International Committee of the Red Cross (ICRC) in Tbilisi, Georgia. In 2010, he deployed to Haiti as a member of the US Department of Health and Human Service's National Disaster Medical System's Disaster Mortuary Operational Response Team (DMORT) to assist with the recovery and identification of earthquake victims. In addition, Dr. Bethard has been involved in bioarchaeological research in the United States, Peru, and the Transylvanian region of Romania. He is a Fellow of the Anthropology Section of the American Academy of Forensic Sciences, a Diplomate of the American Board of Forensic Anthropology, and a Lifetime Member of the American Association of Physical Anthropologists.

**Katelyn L. Bolhofner, PhD,** is currently an Assistant Professor of Physical/Forensic Anthropology at Texas Tech University, where she oversees the Forensic Anthropology Concentration for undergraduate students, supervises graduate students in the Department of Sociology, Anthropology, and Social Work and in the Institute for Forensic Sciences, and through Texas Tech University's Forensic Anthropology Laboratory provides anthropological service to county law enforcement on request. Katelyn received her PhD from Arizona State University was trained in Forensic Anthropology at the Maricopa County Office of the Medical Examiner in Phoenix, Arizona. She continues to collaborate with anthropologists there and at Arizona State University. She has conducted skeletal research in Spain, Cyprus, and on Nubian collections from ancient Sudan and maintains active research agendas in these and other areas.

**Christian Crowder, PhD, D-ABFA** received his BA from Texas A&M University, MA from the University of Texas at Arlington, and PhD from the University of Toronto. He is currently the forensic anthropologist for the Dallas County Medical Examiner's Office in Dallas, Texas. Prior to this he has held the following positions: Director of Forensic Anthropology for the Harris County Institute of Forensic Sciences (HCIFS) in Houston, Texas; chief forensic anthropologist for the Office of the Armed Forces Medical Examiner at Dover AFB; Deputy Director of Forensic Anthropology Unit for the Office of Chief Medical Examiner – New York City; and Forensic Anthropologist for the Defense POW/MIA Accounting Agency (formally the Joint POW/MIA Accounting Command Central Identification Laboratory) in Hawaii. In addition to his practitioner duties, Dr. Crowder is adjunct faculty at Pace University, NYC, and an assistant professor at UT Southwestern Medical Center.

**Elizabeth A. DiGangi, PhD, D-ABFA**, is a bioarchaeologist and forensic anthropologist with research interests in improving trauma analysis and human rights. Currently, she is Assistant Professor of Anthropology at Binghamton University. Prior to this faculty position, she was a contracted forensic science advisor in Colombia, offering a variety of training courses for the country's professional forensic scientists. She continues to mentor and offer courses for forensic scientists in Algeria. It was a research methods course developed by her and a colleague for Colombian anthropologists that led to the publication of her co-edited volume (with Megan Moore): *Research Methods in Human Skeletal Biology* (Academic Press, 2013). She is second author (with Susan Sincerbox) of *Forensic Taphonomy and Ecology of North American Scavengers* (Academic Press, 2018). She works on forensic cases for local and state law enforcement in addition to teaching and mentoring undergraduate and graduate students.

**Julie M. Fleischman, PhD**, is a forensic anthropologist at the Harris County Institute of Forensic Sciences (HCIFS) in Houston, TX. She completed her postdoctoral forensic anthropology fellowship at HCIFS in 2018, and was formerly the laboratory manager for the Michigan State University Forensic Anthropology Laboratory, and an intern at the Maricopa County Office of the Medical Examiner. Her research interests include skeletal trauma and the application of forensic anthropological methods to human rights conflicts, specifically in Cambodia.

**Gary Hodges, BA,** is a litigation graphics specialist at the Maricopa County Attorney's Office in Phoenix, Arizona, where he specializes in creating a wide range of visual aids for use in courtroom presentations – from anatomical illustrations to complex 3D virtual recreations of crime scenes. Mr. Hodges received his bachelor's degree in Anthropology (emphasizing the physical and forensic fields) from Northern Arizona University in 1999. He has certifications in crime scene investigation, police photography, and fingerprint collection and analysis. In addition to his criminal work, he has studied and practiced art his entire life, worked as a freelance writer and graphic designer for over 15 years, and is the creator, writer, and illustrator of his own series of comic books.

**Thomas D. Holland, JD, PhD, RPA, D-ABFA,** is Director of Partnerships and Innovations for the Defense POW/MIA Accounting Agency at the Pentagon. Previously, he directed the Department of Defense Central Identification Laboratory in Hawaii for 23 years, where he was charged with the sole responsibility for identifying the remains of US personnel lost from past military conflicts. While there, he led recovery missions to numerous countries including North Korea, Iraq, Kuwait, China, and Cambodia. He received a Ph.D. in Anthropology from the University of Missouri-Columbia in 1991 and a JD from the University of Hawaii, Richardson School of Law in 2016. He is a Fellow of the American Academy of Forensic Sciences, a Diplomate of the American Board of Forensic Anthropology, and is licensed to practice law in Arkansas and the District of Columbia. He founded the Scientific Working Group for Forensic Anthropology (SWGANTH) and serves, or has served, on numerous committees and advisory groups including the Organization of Scientific Area Committees (OSAC) for Forensic Science, the Department of Justice Crime Scene Committee, the White House Office of Science and Technology's Interagency Group of Forensic Science, and the Forensic Advisory Boards for the International Committee of the Red Cross in Switzerland and the International Commission on Missing Persons in Bosnia. His research interests include prehistoric archeology, evolutionary theory, forensic science, and the intersection of science and the law.

**Jennifer C. Love, PhD, D-ABFA,** is currently the forensic anthropologist and identification unit supervisor for the Office of Chief Medical Examiner (OCME) in Washington, DC. Prior to joining the OCME, she served as the forensic anthropology director at the Harris County Institute of Forensic Sciences in Houston, TX. She is a member of the Anthropology Subcommittee of the Organization for Scientific Area Committees (OSAC). Her research interests are bone trauma, bone pathology, and decedent identification. In 2011, she coauthored the textbook *Skeletal Atlas of Child Abuse*.

**Hon. Daniel Martin** is a Superior Court Judge in Maricopa County. He was appointed to the bench in 2007 and is currently assigned to the civil division, where he presides over complex and commercial matters. Judge Martin received his law degree from the University of Arizona and served as the Managing Editor of the *Arizona Law Review*. Following his graduation, Judge Martin clerked for Justice James Moeller on the Arizona Supreme Court. After seven years in private practice, Judge Martin joined the Office of Administrative Hearings as an Administrative Law Judge, where he served for almost eight years before joining the Superior Court. Prior to his assignment to the civil bench, Judge Martin completed rotations on the family, criminal, and juvenile benches.

**Michal L. Pierce, MS, ASQ CMQ/OE,** received her Bachelor of Science in Microbiology from the University of Illinois, followed by a Master of Science in Forensic Science from Sam Houston State University. She joined the Harris County Institute of Forensic Sciences (HCIFS) Forensic Biology Laboratory in October 2007 as a DNA analyst, and she served as the QA/Compliance Manager for Forensic Genetics from 2011 to 2013. In 2013, she was appointed as the first Quality Director for the HCIFS. In this position, she oversees the Quality Management Division, which includes quality assurance, training and development, and analytical statistics. Ms. Pierce possesses a certification by the American Board of Criminalistics in Molecular Biology, and she is certified as a Manager of Quality/Organizational Excellence through the American Society for Quality.

**Andrew C. Seidel, PhD** received his doctoral degree from Arizona State University, with an emphasis on bioarchaeology. He has published on a number of topics, including the estimation of age-at-death, trauma analysis, and the heritability of traits of the human dentition. His research interests include forensic anthropology, human anatomy and osteology, mortuary analysis, and the archeology of the Eastern Woodlands. Currently, he assists with forensic anthropology casework at the Maricopa County Office of the Medical Examiner.

**Katherine Taylor, PhD, D-ABFA,** is a Forensic Anthropologist with the King County Medical Examiner's Officer where she has worked as a Forensic Anthropologist for over 25 years. As a part of her responsibilities, Dr. Taylor is a lead subject matter expert on mass fatality and victim identification. Dr. Taylor serves on several boards including the Family and Friends of Violent Crime Victims and the Seattle University Criminal Justice Advisory Board. Dr. Taylor is also a Diplomate of the American Board of Forensic Anthropology, a fellow of the American Academy of Forensic Sciences and a member of the Washington Association of Coroners and Medical Examiners. Dr. Taylor is an affiliate faculty at the University of Washington, Department of Anthropology, and an adjunct faculty at the Seattle University Department of Criminal Justice. Dr. Taylor received her PhD in Forensic Anthropology from the University of Arizona.

**Doug Ubelaker, PhD** is a curator and senior scientist at the Smithsonian Institution's National Museum of Natural History in Washington, D.C. where he has been employed for over four decades. Since 1978, he has served as a consultant in forensic anthropology. In this capacity, he has served as an expert witness, reporting on more than 980 cases and has testified in numerous legal proceedings.

He is a Professorial Lecturer with the Departments of Anatomy and Anthropology at the George Washington University, Washington D.C. and is an Adjunct Professor with the Department of Anthropology, Michigan State University, East Lansing, Michigan.

Dr. Ubelaker has published extensively in the general field of human skeletal biology with an emphasis on forensic applications. He has served on the editorial boards of numerous leading scientific publications, including the *Journal of Forensic Sciences; The Open Forensic Science Journal; International Journal of Legal Medicine; Human Evolution; Homo, Journal of Comparative Human Biology; Anthropologie, International Journal of the Science of Man; Forensic Science Communications; Human Evolution; International Journal of Anthropology; Forensic Sciences Research, Forensic Science International*, Science and Justice and *Global Bioethics*.

Dr. Ubelaker received a Bachelor of Arts Degree and a Doctor of Philosophy from the University of Kansas. He has been a member of the American Academy of Forensic Sciences since 1974 and achieved the status of Fellow in 1987 in the Physical Anthropology Section. He served as the 2011–2012 President of the AAFS. He is a Retired Diplomate of the American Board of Forensic Anthropologists.

Dr. Ubelaker has received numerous honors including the Memorial Medal of Dr. Aleš Hrdlička, Humpolec, Czech Republic; the Anthropology Award of the Washington Academy of Sciences; the T. Dale Stewart Award of the Physical Anthropology Section of the American Academy of Forensic Sciences; Distinguished Fellow (2016) and Douglas M. Lucas Medalist (2017) American Academy of Forensic Sciences; the FBI Director's Award for Exceptional Public Service; the Federal Highway Administration Pennsylvania Division Historic Preservation Excellence Award, the Hong Kong Forensic Foundation Award, International Academy of Forensic Sciences and a special recognition award from the FBI. He was elected Miembro Honorario of the Sociedad de Odontoestomatólogos Forenses Ibero Americanos, Profesor Ad Honorem, Universidad de la República, Facultad de Medicina, Montevideo, Uruguay, Socio Honorario, Asociación Latinoaméricana de Antropologia Forense, Honoris Causa FASE certification, Milano, Italy and Doctor (Honoris Causa) University of Cordoba, Argentina.

**Lauren Zephro, PhD**, is currently the laboratory director for the Santa Cruz County Sheriff's Office Forensic Services Division. She earned her MA from the University of Tennessee, Knoxville, and her PhD from the University of California, Santa Cruz. In addition to her work as a forensic anthropologist, she is also a fingerprint expert and specializes in crime scene investigation. She is a Fellow of the Anthropology Section of the American Academy of Forensic Sciences and a Certified Latent Print Examiner through the International Association for Identification. Her research interests include bone trauma, bone biomechanics and secular change in skeletal morphology.

# Preface

The criterion separating Forensic Anthropologists from other Anthropologists or Archeologists is that they operate within the realm of the medico-legal system. One definition of the term "forensic" means relating to or dealing with the application of scientific knowledge to legal problems. In the context of this volume the authors are discussing the application of scientific knowledge as it pertains to anthropology casework performed in the legal milieu.

Forensic Anthropology has its roots in Biological or Physical Anthropology. Much of the methodological underpinnings of the science were developed for use on dissection cadavers or on skeletons derived from archeological contexts. The application of these scientific principles to forensic casework began organically as consultations to local academicians and slowly morphed into the varied and dynamic field of study observed today.

As Forensic Anthropology developed somewhat accidentally, there are no hard and fast training tenets for one of the outcomes of forensic casework, namely interaction with the judicial system. Anthropologists are left to either figure it out on their own, or observe other practitioners such as forensic pathologists or forensic toxicologists, who testify on a more routine basis. This kind of on the job training does not suffice when a legal proceeding is particularly complex or multi-layered.

This volume was developed to address that basic gap in the training of most Forensic Anthropologists. The content is divided into two conceptual parts: the first (Chapters 1–4) is an historical overview and current state of the field as it is today; the second (Chapters 5–12) is meant to be used as a hands-on manual designed to provide basic, essential information that will assist practitioners facing legal proceedings.

The editors of this volume are seasoned professionals who each bring a unique perspective to the work. Our hope is that we have covered the multi-faceted aspects of the United States Judicial System and provided meaningful information about its vagaries. Many of the legal terms used in the volume are defined in the accompanying glossary, or in the text where they are found. Legal procedures are defined and explained. The entire process is laid out and discussed from varying perspectives in an attempt to provide clarity about the expectations of the legal community regarding forensic scientists. While the book is geared toward Forensic Anthropology our hope is that any forensic scientist could gain insight from the information presented.

The authors contributing to this volume present material in their particular area of expertise. In Chapter 1, Love and Fulginiti cover the constitutional underpinnings of the Confrontation Clause and how it applies to Forensic Science. Chapter 1 is followed by a detailed discussion by Holland and Crowder of the historical events leading up to the issuance of the 2009 National Academy of Science (NAS) report and its impact on forensic science. This report was extremely critical of the way in which forensic science is performed and regulated and became a harbinger of significant change. In Chapter 2, these authors discuss the imperative for reliable research to uphold anthropological methods.

Following on that discussion, Bethard and DiGangi tackle research developments in the field by assessing the *Journal of Forensic Sciences* and discuss the implications of research in the legal milieu. The final chapter in this part of the volume is written by newly fledged PhDs, Bolhofner and Seidel, who discuss the current state of Forensic Anthropology training programs from the perspective of individuals who have recently navigated those waters. Combined, these first chapters represent the section of the volume designed to introduce the reader to the medico-legal community and define the place of Forensic Anthropology expert witnesses in it.

The second part of the volume, beginning with Chapter 5, transitions into a "how-to" manual for professionals currently practicing, and for students who are considering Forensic Anthropology as a career. The first chapter in this section, by Fleischman et al., straddles the two parts of the volume by presenting the background and history around quality assurance and control in a forensic laboratory while also presenting details regarding how to go about setting up a laboratory and if desired pursuing accreditation for that laboratory. Fleischman et al. detail the importance of a strong QA/QC program in any Forensic Anthropology laboratory and in forensic casework.

The next chapters, by Zephro and Galloway, detail the recommended documentation, both written and photographic, that should be maintained from the beginning of any accepted forensic case. The authors present important information regarding the kinds of material to consider putting into a case report, what to maintain in the case file, and how to document the case effectively so that another practitioner could understand every step that was taken and how conclusions were engendered. Hartnett-McCann et al. present an argument for the importance of a robust peer review process; their chapter both explains how to develop one and emphasizes the necessity of this practice in every Forensic Anthropology caseload. Forensic Anthropology as a discipline is becoming a more integral part of the medico-legal system and our procedures must conform to best practices.

The final chapters in the book, Chapters 9–12, focus on interaction with the legal community, beginning with a detailed description of the United States

Judicial System. Martin and Fulginiti outline many of the pre-trial proceedings and documents and explain them in the context of an expert witness. The expectations of the Court are laid out and courtroom etiquette is described. Chapter 9 contains critical information for practitioners facing legal proceedings as an expert.

Hodges, in Chapter 10, describes the field of litigation graphics; how to go about best presenting your findings so that a lay jury can understand them more easily. He also uses a case study to demonstrate the effectiveness of good graphics when communicating complex scientific principles. Building on this example, Hodges underscores the importance of clear communication in the courtroom.

Bartelink et al., in Chapter 11, provide a pertinent discussion of the interactions among expert witnesses in what is essentially an adversarial system. The authors provide support for maintaining independence in casework, case management and critically, expert testimony. In the final chapter, Galloway et al. detail the importance of placing a fair market value on your professional time. The authors provide examples and useful suggestions regarding how to track and bill cases. Forensic Anthropologists often have a difficult time placing a value on work they consider to be a service to the community and Chapter 12 addresses such issues.

The chapter appendices and glossary are meant to provide examples of different types of documents as well as define unfamiliar legal jargon. The hope of the editors is that this volume presents timely and detailed meaningful information that can be used to train new practitioners, to provide a path for scientists who have not yet testified, and to clarify the various procedures for even battle-weary experts.

**Fulgi, Kristen, and Alison**

# Series preface

The forensic sciences represent diverse, dynamic fields that seek to utilize the very best techniques available to address legal issues. Fueled by advances in technology, research and methodology, as well as new case applications, the forensic sciences continue to evolve. Forensic scientists strive to improve their analyses and interpretations of evidence and to remain cognizant of the latest advancements. This series results from a collaborative effort between the American Academy of Forensic Sciences (AAFS) and Wiley to publish a select number of books that relate closely to the activities and Objectives of the AAFS. The book series reflects the goals of the AAFS to encourage quality scholarship and publication in the forensic sciences. Proposals for publication in the series are reviewed by a committee established for that purpose by the AAFS and also reviewed by Wiley. The AAFS was founded in 1948 and represents a multidisciplinary professional organization that provides leadership to advance science and its application to the legal system. The 11 sections of the AAFS consist of Criminalistics, Digital and Multimedia Sciences, Engineering Sciences, General, Pathology/Biology, Questioned Documents, Jurisprudence, Anthropology, Toxicology, Odontology, and Psychiatry and Behavioral Science. There are over 7000 members of the AAFS, originating from all 50 States of the United States and many countries beyond. This series reflects global AAFS membership interest in new research, scholarship, and publication in the forensic sciences.

**Douglas H. Ubelaker**
Senior Scientist
Smithsonian Institution
Washington, DC, USA
Series Editor

# Foreword

The rapidly expanding field of Forensic Anthropology involves the application of anthropological methodology to medico-legal issues. Students and colleagues entering this academic discipline must learn techniques of detection and recovery, species recognition, evaluation of the biological profile, estimating time since death and detecting evidence of trauma and post-mortem modifications. Training for this analysis is largely available in educational programs related to bioarcheology, skeletal biology and related academic foci. However, those working in Forensic Anthropology must also master techniques unique to forensic applications, especially in regards to trauma analysis and evaluation of the post-mortem interval. The medico-legal context presents other challenges for the Forensic Anthropologist. Results of analysis must be presented properly in the judicial system. The Forensic Anthropologist must be prepared for the possibility of court testimony and/or deposition. Preparation involves not only assembling bench notes, reports, and aspects of documentation, but also understanding the legal process and what is expected of the involved scientist. This new book provides welcomed perspective regarding the legal context of the work of Forensic Anthropology.

This volume focuses on forensic applications within the judicial systems of North America. In this area of the world, courts depend upon the adversary process and cross-examination to maintain the quality of scientific testimony (Peterson and Murdock 1989). In recent years, concern regarding the science presented in the legal system has led to evidentiary standards (Christensen and Crowder 2009) that must be understood by Forensic Anthropologists and others in forensic science. Forensic Anthropologists must be competent and meet broader ethical standards as well (Peterson and Murdock 1989).

Growing numbers of Forensic Anthropologists apply their skills in countries other than their own (Kranioti and Paine 2011; Rosenblatt 2010). Such involvement reflects the global expansion of the field of Forensic Anthropology, as well as the many applications to humanitarian and human rights issues (Cattaneo 2007; Cattaneo and Baccino 2002; Doretti and Snow 2003; Fleischman 2016; Işcan and Olivera 2000; Klinkner 2008; Steadman and Haglund 2005; Sikkink 2008; Stover and Ryan 2001; Ubelaker 2008). Many of the issues relating to scientific testimony are universal. All systems recognize the need for well-trained and competent scientific testimony and the importance of proper recovery and documentation of evidence (Crossland 2013; Haglund 2001; Hanson 2008; Schmitt 2002). However, the legal context also presents considerable global diversity (Ubelaker 2015). International law relating to scientific testimony reflects local culture, values, history, and traditions (Merry 1992, 2006). Many countries, especially in Europe adhere to the adversarial system with cross-examination that also is employed in North America. Others utilize the inquisitorial system with its focus on balance maintained by the prosecutor (Ubelaker 2015). Some differences even exist in forensic-related law between the United States and Canada (Holobinko 2012).

Forensic Anthropologists working globally also need to become aware of international humanitarian and human rights law. The United Nations has established International Tribunals for the prosecution of serious violations of international humanitarian laws. These include the International Criminal Tribunal for the former Yugoslavia (ICTY) and a similar one for Rwanda (ICTR) (Cordner and McKelvie 2002). Many anthropologists have conducted analyses in association with these tribunals and the violations they address (Baraybar and Gasior 2006; Fondebrider 2015; Kimmerle and Baraybar 2008; Kimmerle and Jantz 2008; Klinkner 2009; Komar 2003; Stover and Shigekane 2002).

Clearly, the legal context of the work of Forensic Anthropologists is complex and challenging to comprehend. This volume clarifies many of the issues involved to assist Forensic Anthropologists in their involvement with the legal system. It provides guidelines relating to the judicial system that need to be considered during the entire process of forensic activity from data recovery to court testimony. Forensic Anthropologists, especially those entering the field, need to understand what is expected of them from the legal system. This new book provides that important information.

**Douglas H. Ubelaker**

# References

Baraybar, J.P. and Gasior, M. (2006). Forensic anthropology and the most probable cause of death in cases of violations against international humanitarian law: an example from Bosnia and Herzegovina. *Journal of Forensic Sciences* 51 (1): 103–108.

Cattaneo, C. (2007). Forensic anthropology: developments of a classical discipline in the new millennium. *Forensic Science International* 165 (2): 185–193.

Cattaneo, C. and Baccino, E. (2002). A call for forensic anthropology in Europe. *International Journal of Legal Medicine* 116 (6): N1–N2.

Christensen, A.M. and Crowder, C.M. (2009). Evidentiary standards for forensic anthropology. *Journal of Forensic Sciences* 54 (6): 1211–1216.

Cordner, S. and McKelvie, H. (2002). Developing standards in international forensic work to identify missing persons. *International Review of the Red Cross* 84 (848): 867–884.

Crossland, Z. (2013). Evidential regimes of forensic anthropology. *Annual Review of Anthropology* 42 (1): 121–137.

Doretti, M. and Snow, C.C. (2003). Forensic anthropology and human rights: the Argentine experience. In: *Hard Evidence: Case Studies in Forensic Anthropology* (ed. D.W. Steadman), 290–310. Upper Saddle River, NJ: Pearson Education.

Fleischman, J.M. (2016). Working with the remains in Cambodia: skeletal analysis and human rights after atrocity. *Genocide Studies and Prevention: An International Journal* 10 (2): 121–130.

Fondebrider, L. (2015). Forensic anthropology and the investigation of political violence: lessons learned from Latin American and the Balkans. In: *Necropolitics: Mass Graves and Exhumations in the Age of Human Rights* (ed. F. Ferrándiz and A.C.G.M. Robben), 41–52. Philadelphia, PA: University of Pennsylvania Press.

Haglund, W.D. (2001). Archaeology and forensic death investigations. *Historical Archaeology* 35 (1): 26–34.

Hanson, I. (2008). Forensic archaeology: approaches to international investigations. In: *Forensic Approaches to Death, Disaster and Abuse* (ed. M. Oxenham), 1–12. Sydney: Australian Academic Press.

Holobinko, A. (2012). Forensic human identification in the United States and Canada: a review of the law, admissible techniques, and the legal implications of their application in forensic cases. *Forensic Science International* 222: 394.e1–394.e13.

İşcan, M.Y. and Olivera, H.E.S. (2000). Forensic anthropology in Latin America. *Forensic Science International* 109: 15–30.

Kimmerle, E.H. and Baraybar, J.P. (eds.) (2008). An epidemiological approach to forensic investigations of violations to international humanitarian and human rights law. In: *Skeletal Trauma: Identification of Injuries Resulting from Human Rights and Abuse and Armed Conflict*, 1–13. Boca Raton, FL: CRC Press.

Kimmerle, E.H. and Jantz, R.L. (2008). Variation as evidence: introduction to a symposium on international human identification. *Journal of Forensic Sciences* 53 (3): 521–523.

Klinkner, M. (2008). Forensic science for Cambodian justice. *The International Journal for Transitional Justice* 2 (2): 227–243.

Klinkner, M. (2009). Forensic science expertise for international criminal proceedings: an old problem, a new context and a pragmatic resolution. *The International Journal of Evidence & Proof* 13 (2): 102–129.

Komar, D. (2003). Lessons from Srebrenica: the contributions and limitations of physical anthropology in identifying victims of war crimes. *Journal of Forensic Sciences* 48 (4): 713–716.

Kranioti, E.F. and Paine, R.R. (2011). Forensic anthropology in Europe: an assessment of current status and application. *Journal of Anthropological Sciences* 89: 71–92.

Merry, S.E. (1992). Anthropology, law, and transnational processes. *Annual Review of Anthropology* 21: 357–379.

Merry, S.E. (2006). Anthropology and international law. *Annual Review of Anthropology* 35: 99–116.

Peterson, J.L. and Murdock, J.E. (1989). Forensic science ethics: developing an integrated system of support and enforcement. *Journal of Forensic Sciences* 34 (3): 749–762.

Rosenblatt, A. (2010). International forensic investigations and the human rights of the dead. *Human Rights Quarterly* 32 (4): 921–950.

Schmitt, S. (2002). Mass graves and the collection of forensic evidence: genocide, war crimes, and crimes against humanity. In: *Advances in Forensic Taphonomy: Method, Theory, and Archaeological Perspectives* (ed. W.D. Haglund and M.H. Sorg), 277–291. Boca Raton, FL: CRC Press.

Sikkink, K. (2008). From pariah state to global protagonist: Argentina and the struggle for international human rights. *Latin American Politics and Society* 50 (1): 1–29.

Steadman, D.W. and Haglund, W.D. (2005). The scope of anthropological contributions to human rights investigations. *Journal of Forensic Sciences* 50 (1): 23–30.

Stover, E. and Ryan, M. (2001). Breaking bread with the dead. *Historical Archaeology* 35 (1): 7–25.

Stover, E. and Shigekane, R. (2002). The missing in the aftermath of war: when do the needs of victims' families and international war crimes tribunals clash? *International Review of the Red Cross* 84 (848): 845–866.

Ubelaker, D.H. (2008). Issues in the global applications of methodology in forensic anthropology. *Journal of Forensic Sciences* 53 (3): 606–607.

Ubelaker, D.H. (ed.) (2015). *The Global Practice of Forensic Science*. Chichester: Wiley Blackwell.

# Acknowledgments

The editors would like to express their appreciation for Wiley Publishing and especially for Jenny Cossham and Adalfin Jayasingh. All editors dread the process of bringing an edited volume into the world but these individuals made the process almost effortless. We highly recommend the Forensic Science in Focus series to anyone with an interest in publication in this arena.

The editors would like to acknowledge the input and subject matter expertise provided by our legal reviewer. He provided oversight, masterful editing and prevented us from falling into a legal quagmire from which there was no rescue. He should have been added as an editor but he declined.

The editors would also like to thank our final reviewers, Drs. Jennifer Love and Katherine Taylor and Daniel J. Martin, esq. They provided important feedback, editing, and clarification that improved the volume significantly.

The editors would like to acknowledge contributor Gary Hodges, Litigation Graphics Specialist, for providing additional figures to enhance the overall text.

The editors would like to acknowledge the commitment and promptness of all of the contributors. Each brought a unique voice to the volume and consequently made it a stronger part of the Forensic Anthropology literature.

Fulgi would like to express gratitude to Dr. Ubelaker and her co-editors: to Doug for showing the way, to Baby Bones for prying open the door and holding it open for others and for being steadfast under all conditions, and to Alison for providing unwavering friendship and support. She would like to thank the Forensic Anthropology community for providing her with a life-long passion filled with fun and engaging colleagues. She recognizes her mentors, J. Michael, Walt, Alison, Mike F., Doug U., John G. and Joe B., and her TB sisters. She is eternally grateful for her Ducklings and to her teaching partner for making her a stronger, more competent practitioner. Most of all Fulgi recognizes her husband Dan, and son Daniel, for their love, support, and input into everything she does. Thank you.

Kristen would like to thank Fulgi and Alison for the opportunity to edit this volume with them. She never imagined she could be in such incredible company. A million thanks to Mama Bones for being an amazing mentor, colleague, and friend. Finally, thanks to John, Owen, and Maddie, for their love, support, and understanding.

Alison would like to thank those who guided her into this field, most especially the late Dr. Walt Birkby and to Dr. M.E. Morbeck who made sure that she actually finished the doctorate. Alison also wants to thank those who made sure that she kept current with practices – her students (Vicki Wedel, Chelsey Juarez, Cris Hughes, and, of course, Lauren Zephro). My daughter, Gwyneth, has picked up a good share of the chores at home while I worked on this volume.

We also owe a debt to the decedents whose bodies we examine, from whom we learn and for whom we continue to strive to improve our work.

# About the editors

**Laura C. Fulginiti** is a Forensic Anthropologist in Maricopa County. She has lived and worked in Phoenix, AZ since 1991. She trained with Dr. Walter Birkby at the University of Arizona after being sent there by Dr. J. Michael Hoffman at The Colorado College. Both men saw her passion and did their best to augment it. Dr. Fulginiti is a subject matter expert in mass fatality response, search and recovery and bone trauma interpretation. She has participated in multiple federal mass victim recovery and identification events including the 9–11 terrorist attacks and Hurricane Katrina. She is a Diplomate of the American Board of Forensic Anthropology and a Fellow of the American Academy of Forensic Sciences (AAFS). She currently serves as the Vice President of AAFS and as a Trustee for the Forensic Sciences Foundation. She lives with her husband and three cats. They have a son, Daniel, who in spite of her best efforts chose to be an attorney instead of a scientist. She might have exposed him to forensics a little too early.

**Kristen Hartnett-McCann** is a board-certified Forensic Anthropologist at the Office of the Chief Medical Examiner in Farmington, CT, where she performs forensic anthropological casework and scene response. Prior to her employment in CT, she was the Assistant Director of Forensic Anthropology at the Office of Chief Medical Examiner in New York City (NYC). While in NYC, she was active in casework and participated in the recovery and identification efforts at the World Trade Center. She is also the consulting forensic anthropologist for Suffolk County on Long Island as well as other counties in New York. In addition, she is an adjunct professor at Hofstra University, is an appointed member of the Crime Scene/Death Investigation Scientific Area Committee (SAC) Anthropology Subcommittee, within the Organization of Scientific Area Committees (OSAC) under the National Institute of Standards and Technology (NIST), and is the Co-vice Chair of the Academy Standards Board (ASB) Anthropology Consensus Body. Her research and applied interests include the estimation of age and sex from the adult skeleton, taphonomy, blunt and sharp force trauma, expert witness testimony, crime scene response, and mass disaster preparedness/response. She lives in Long Island, NY, with her husband, John, and their two children, Owen and Madeline.

**Alison Galloway** is Professor Emerita of Anthropology at the University of California, Santa Cruz. She is a board-certified Forensic Anthropologist and a Fellow of the American Academy of Forensic Sciences. Initially trained as an archeologist at UC Berkeley, she moved to forensic anthropology during her graduate work at the University of Arizona, studying with Dr. Walter Birkby. Her forensic research has focused on the postmortem interval, skeletal damage produced by fire and the legal/ethic context of forensic anthropology. She is co-editor of two books, *The Evolving Female* and *Broken Bones: Anthropological Analysis of Blunt Force Trauma*. She is an active consultant for a number of jurisdictions in the central sections of California and also has consulted frequently for the defense. She lives in Amador County, CA with her dogs and horses.

# Glossary

**ABFA (American Board of Forensic Anthropology) certification**
Professional certification in Forensic Anthropology that denotes the highest recognized level of qualification in the discipline and based on a qualifying examination, a personal and professional record of education and training, experience, and achievement.

**Accreditation** Exists to set minimum requirements for those practicing in the same field and ultimately leads to some sense of uniformity between different agencies. Accreditation is for a service, not a person. Laboratory accreditation embodies not just the practitioners themselves, but also the infrastructure within which they work, including the quality management system.

**Administrative review** Ensures that the record is complete, uses correct spelling and grammar, is properly classified, and complies with laboratory requirements and practices.

**Affidavit** A sworn statement for use in legal proceedings.

**Arraign/arraignment** Court hearing in a criminal case during which the charges are read out to the accused, and he or she must plead guilty or not guilty.

**Bench notes** Notes recorded during laboratory analysis.

**Calibration** A set of operations that establish, under specified conditions, the relationship between values of quantities indicated by a measuring instrument or measuring system, or values represented by a material measure or a reference material, and the corresponding values realized by the standards.

**Chain of custody** The chronological documentation recording the sequence of custody, control, transfer, analysis, and disposition of evidence (both physical and electronic).

**Cognitive bias** The tendency to perceive information based on one's own experiences and preferences.

**Common law** Body of written court decisions; a rule of law established by a higher court. Also known as precedent.

**Competency** Observable and measurable knowledge, skills, or abilities that contribute to enhanced performance and ultimately result in organizational success.

**Compulsory Process Clause** In the Sixth Amendment of the US Constitution, it enables a defendant to subpoena a witness and to force him/her to testify.

**Confirmation bias** The tendency to interpret new information/evidence as validation of one's existing beliefs.

**Confrontation Clause** The Confrontation Clause compels the witness "to stand face to face with the jury in order that they may look at him, and judge by his demeanor upon the stand and the manner in which he gives his testimony whether he is worthy of belief." (*Mattox v. United States*, 1895, Section 3, para. 4). The Clause requires prosecution witnesses to testify under oath and subjects them to cross-examination. The witnesses must testify in court in the presence of the defendant. The Clause also guarantees the defendant's right to be present in the courtroom throughout the trial.

**Cross-examination** The questioning of a witness, called to testify at a trial or hearing, by the opposing party.

**D-ABFA** Diplomate of the ABFA. The designation of a person who has been awarded board certified in Forensic Anthropology through the ABFA (American Board of Forensic Anthropology).

*Daubert* **hearing** An evaluation by a trial judge on the admissibility of expert testimony or evidence. This hearing is conducted outside the jury's presence and usually occurs before the trial begins.

**Defense/defendant** The side of a legal case that is sued or accused in a court of law.

**Deposition** A formal interview conducted under oath in the presence of a court reporter that results in a transcript of the deponent's sworn testimony.

**Direct examination** The questioning of a witness at a trial or hearing by the side who called the witness to testify.

**Discoverable** Documents, Evidence, Witness statements, etc. that must be disclosed to the opposite side in legal proceedings.

**Discovery** The investigation and information gathering stage of litigation. Each party in legal proceedings can obtain evidence from the other party or parties.

**Expert witness** A person who is allowed to testify at a trial because of special knowledge or proficiency in a particular field, beyond that of the ordinary lay person.

**Forensic anthropologist** A biological anthropologist with specialized training in the analysis of skeletal remains and interpretation of osseous traumata, pathologic conditions, skeletal variants, and postmortem interval in a medico-legal context.

*Frye* **hearing** A hearing held to determine the admissibility of scientific evidence or expert testimony.

**Grand jury** A group of people (usually 23 in the US) selected to examine the validity of an accusation before trial.

**Indictment**   A formal charge or accusation.

**Inquest**   A judicial inquiry to find out the facts relating to an incident, such as a death.

**Internal validation**   The methods and equipment being used are working properly in a specific laboratory, and that personnel are properly trained and qualified to use such methods and equipment in said laboratory. Also uses "knowns" as verification.

**Jury**   A group of people (typically 8 or 12 in the US) sworn to give a verdict in a legal case on the basis of evidence submitted to them in court.

**KUMHO TIRE v. Carmichael**   The Supreme Court sought to strengthen trial courts' roles as gatekeepers of scientific testimony in *Daubert v. Merrell Dow Pharmaceuticals, Inc.*, 509 U.S. 579 (1993). After *Daubert*, many practitioners believed that the new "*Daubert* standard" for admissibility only applied to scientific expert testimony. But in *Kumho Tire v. Carmichael*, 526 U.S. 137 (1999), the Supreme Court held that the Daubert standard applies to all expert opinions under Evidence Rule 702, clarifying that, whether a forensic expert is considered a "scientist" or a "technician," their testimony must be evaluated under *Daubert*.

**Lay witness**   A person who testifies based upon their personal knowledge and life experiences. A lay witness is different to an expert witness because an expert witness testifies based on their qualifications and expertise in a particular field.

**Peer review**   The evaluation of scientific, academic, or professional work by someone working in the same field.

**Plaintiff**   A person or entity who brings a claim against another in a court of law.

**Plan-do-check-act (PDCA) cycle**   The most common model for improving quality. The steps of this cycle include: (i) plan the intended change by deciding what actions are needed to achieve the change; (ii) perform the actions to carry out the change, either in a pilot program or on a small scale; (iii) assess the results and effectiveness of the changes; and (iv) proceed accordingly.

**Post-conviction relief**   A legal process that takes place after a trial that results in the conviction of a defendant, whereby the convicted person can request that a sentence be corrected or vacated.

**Precedent**   Body of written court decisions; a rule of law established by a higher court. Also known as common law.

**Proficiency/proficient**   A high degree of competence, skill, or expertise.

**Pro bono**   From the Latin phrase, "pro bono publico," meaning "for the public good." Usually refers to services offered without taking a fee.

**Prosecution/prosecutor**    The legal proceedings against an individual accused of a crime and the attorney responsible for carrying it out.

**Public defender**    An attorney provided by the government in a criminal trial to represent a defendant who cannot afford their own counsel.

**Quality assurance**    Ensures that processes are conducive for generating a quality product or service.

**Quality control**    A process that focuses on testing the conformity of a product or service.

**Quality management**    The planning and policy-making of top management to support quality control, quality assurance, and quality improvement initiatives.

**Redirect examination**    The additional direct examination of a witness following cross-examination.

**Sixth Amendment**    Found in the US Constitution. "In all criminal prosecutions, the accused shall enjoy the right to a speedy and public trial, by an impartial jury of the State and district wherein the crime shall have been committed, which district shall have been previously ascertained by law, and to be informed of the nature and cause of the accusation; to be confronted with the witnesses against him; to have compulsory process for obtaining witnesses in his favor, and to have the Assistance of Counsel for his defense." The Sixth Amendment was passed by Congress on September 25, 1789 and ratified on December 15, 1791. The purpose of the Sixth Amendment was to legitimize criminal prosecution ensuring accuracy and fairness.

**Standard operating procedures (SOPs)**    A set of step-by-step instructions compiled by an organization to help workers carry out routine operations. The goals of an SOP are to inform staff regarding the proper way to carry out a task, and to establish a minimum level of uniformity among the staff when carrying out the same activity.

**Subpoena**    An order or summons for a person to compel their attendance in court.

**Supremacy Clause**    Article VI in the US Constitution; establishes that the US Constitution, federal laws, and treaties made under its authority, constitute the supreme law of the land. In cases where there is conflict between federal and state law, the federal law must be applied.

**Technical review**    Evaluates notes, data, and other supporting records that form the basis of the scientific results and conclusions contained in the report. The technical review consists of determining whether the appropriate examinations have been performed, the conclusions are consistent with the recorded data, and are within the scope of the discipline and/or category of testing.

**Validation**  An assessment of either a method or piece of equipment to determine whether its efficacy and reliability meet the requirements specified for its use in the laboratory.

**Verification**  An assessment of whether a method or procedure can be followed or applied adequately within the laboratory once validated.

*Voir dire*  A preliminary examination or hearing of a witness or juror by a judge or counsel.

**PART I**
# Context

# CHAPTER 1

# Confrontation: where forensic science meets the sixth amendment

Jennifer C. Love[1] and Laura C. Fulginiti[2]

[1] *District of Columbia Office of the Medical Examiner, Washington, DC, USA*
[2] *Maricopa County, Office of the Medical Examiner, Phoenix, AZ, USA*

"There are few subjects, perhaps, upon which this Court and other courts have been more nearly unanimous than in their expressions of belief that the right of confrontation and cross-examination is an essential and fundamental requirement for the kind of fair trial which is this country's constitutional goal." (Pointer v Texas, 1965, Section I, para.4).

The Confrontation Clause compels the witness "to stand face to face with the jury in order that they may look at him, and judge by his demeanor upon the stand and the manner in which he gives his testimony whether he is worthy of belief." (Mattox v United States, 1895, Section 3, para. 4).

Several United States (US) Supreme Court rulings, framed by the Confrontation Clause of the Sixth Amendment, have spoken directly to the admissibility of forensic analysis and the testimony of forensic scientists. The Confrontation Clause requires criminal defendants to have an opportunity to cross-examine witnesses against them. When the witness is an expert, like a Forensic Anthropologist, their reports can be considered "out-of-court testimony," which means the expert has to appear in court and the defendant has to have an opportunity to question them. Supreme Court rulings on the Confrontation Clause have held that an opportunity for cross-examination is required even if the reports are considered to be reliable (*Crawford v. Washington*, 541 U.S. 36 (2004)), classified forensic analytical reports as out-of-court testimony subject to this requirement, (*Melendez-Diaz v. Massachusetts*, 557 U.S. 305 (2009)), and limited the use of surrogate witnesses to meet this requirement (*Bullcoming v. New Mexico*, 564 U.S. 647 (2011)). But the Supreme Court has so far failed to define who must be called to testify when admitting complex analyses involving several analysts (*Williams v.*

*Forensic Anthropology and the United States Judicial System*, First Edition.
Edited by Laura C. Fulginiti, Kristen Hartnett-McCann, and Alison Galloway.
© 2019 John Wiley & Sons Ltd. Published 2019 by John Wiley & Sons Ltd.

*Illinois*, 567 U.S. 50 (2012)). In these rulings, the US Supreme Court responded to specific case facts set before it and provided guidance for the case at hand. Collaterally, however, these decisions have a ripple effect throughout the legal system, impacting cases with similar but not identical facts, creating significant room for interpretation and at times causing confusion for the lower courts. Furthermore, the Court issued contradicting rulings in two cases addressing the testimony of forensic analysts (*Bullcoming v. New Mexico*, *Williams v. Illinois*). These piecemeal rulings leave prosecutors, defendants, and judges to navigate complex forensic analyses that involve multiple analysts with little direction, catching forensic scientists in the turbulence. Forensic practitioners must be aware of these US Supreme Court decisions, understand their impact on the admissibility of forensic reports, and prepare their laboratory practice to meet the requirements of the legal system.

In this chapter, the US Supreme Court opinions that impact forensic practitioners are presented in chronological order. Some of the cases (*Melendez-Diaz v. Massachusetts*, *Bullcoming v. New Mexico*, *Williams v. Illinois*) directly address admissibility of forensic analytical reports and analyst testimony, while others (*Ohio v. Roberts*, 448 U.S. 56 (1980), *Crawford v. Washington*) provide historical background. Before the court cases are presented, the history of the Sixth Amendment and its importance to the legal system are reviewed. After the court cases, the impact of the Court's opinions on the practice of forensic science is discussed and suggestions for best practice to insure the admissibility of forensic analysis are presented.

## 1.1 Sixth amendment

In all criminal prosecutions, the accused shall enjoy the right to a speedy and public trial, by an impartial jury of the State and district wherein the crime shall have been committed, which district shall have been previously ascertained by law, and to be informed of the nature and cause of the accusation; to be confronted with the witnesses against him; to have compulsory process for obtaining witnesses in his favor, and to have the Assistance of Counsel for his defense.

The Sixth Amendment was passed by Congress on September 25, 1789 and ratified on December 15, 1791 (Bibas and Fisher n.d.). The purpose of the Sixth Amendment was to legitimize criminal prosecution ensuring accuracy and fairness. At the time the Founding Fathers conceived the Bill of Rights, law was maintained by local sheriffs and unsworn men serving as constables or night watchmen. Typically, criminal cases were initiated by an accuser, not a public prosecutor. The accuser and defendant met in trial with no legal counsel, representing themselves and bringing forth witnesses to support their stories.

Trials were short sessions (minutes to hours) of arguing in front of a 12-member jury made up of local citizens who knew both the accuser and the accused. The jurors observed both the accuser and the accused throughout the trial, debated if the defendant was guilty and decided if he deserved mercy. Following the government's power to punish, the jury identified the appropriate punishment, including the death penalty. The process assured the community that justice was carried out swiftly, impartially, and fairly (Bibas and Fisher n.d.). The Sixth Amendment strengthened the adversarial process and maintained the process of each side conducting its own investigation, presenting its own evidence and arguing its side in open court.

The Compulsory Process Clause and the Confrontation Clause directly address the witness as well as the defendant. The Compulsory Process Clause enables a defendant to subpoena a witness and to force him to testify. The Confrontation Clause requires prosecution witnesses to testify under oath and subjects them to cross-examination. The witnesses must testify in court in the presence of the defendant. The Clauses also guarantee the defendant's right to be present in the courtroom throughout the trial (Bibas and Fisher n.d.).

Since the Sixth Amendment was ratified, the practice of law enforcement and the legal system has evolved. Professional police forces became responsible for investigating crimes and arresting suspects. Public prosecutors initiated legal proceedings and defendants hired lawyers to represent them. In some communities, public defender offices were created. Judges created rules of evidence and provided clear instructions to juries. Meanwhile, lawyers began selecting jurors. Trials grew longer and became more complex (Bibas and Fisher n.d.).

By the middle of the nineteenth century, the Supreme Court had ruled that the Sixth Amendment protections applied to state courts as well as federal, greatly expanding the reach of the Amendment. As a result, the Court has had multiple occasions to define the Amendment's protections.

### 1.1.1   *Ohio v. Roberts*, 448 U.S. 56 (1980). Argued November 26, 1979 – decided June 23, 1980

On January 7, 1975, Herschel Roberts was arrested and charged with forgery of checks in the name of Bernard Isaacs and possession of stolen credit cards belonging to Bernard Isaacs. A preliminary hearing was held in Municipal Court. The defense called Anita Isaacs, Bernard Isaacs' daughter, as their only witness. Anita testified that she knew the respondent and that she allowed him to use her apartment while she was away. Defense counsel questioned Anita at length in an attempt to have Anita admit that she gave the checks and credit cards to the respondent without informing him that she did not have permission to use them. Anita denied the allegation. The defense counsel did not ask to have the witness declared hostile nor request permission to cross-examine her. The prosecutor did not question Anita.

Between the preliminary hearing and the trial, five subpoenas for four trial dates were issued to Anita and sent to her parents' address. Anita was not at the address at the time the subpoenas were delivered and she did not appear for trial.

During the trial, Roberts testified that Anita provided him the checks and credit cards with the understanding that he could use them. Following Ohio state law which allows preliminary examination testimony of a witness who cannot for any reason be produced at the trial, the prosecution offered the transcript from Anita's testimony as a rebuttal. The defense objected to the use of the transcript under the Confrontation Clause of the Sixth Amendment. A *voir dire* hearing (a preliminary questioning of a witness to determine his competence to testify) was held and Anita's mother testified that she did not know her daughter's whereabouts, had spoken to her daughter on two occasions since the preliminary hearing, and did not know of anyone who knew her whereabouts. One of the phone conversations with Anita was facilitated by a social worker in San Francisco following a welfare application filed by Anita. The jury found the respondent guilty on all counts.

The Court of Appeals of Ohio reversed the finding on the basis that the prosecution failed to make a showing of "good faith effort" to find the witness. The State made no effort to find the daughter prior to trial; no one attempted to contact the social worker. The only effort made regarding Anita's whereabouts was the *voir dire* requested by the defense.

The Ohio Supreme Court upheld the Court of Appeals ruling, but based on different grounds. Anita's whereabouts were unknown and the trial judge could have reasonably concluded based on Anita's mother's *voir dire* hearing that efforts to find the witness would have been unsuccessful. However, the Court upheld that the transcript was inadmissible on the basis that the respondent did not have an opportunity to cross-examine the witness. The defense had an opportunity to question Anita during the preliminary hearing, but the purpose of the preliminary hearing is to determine probable cause. The Court felt that the mere opportunity to cross-examine a witness did not meet the Confrontation Clause requirement. The fact that the respondent did not cross-examine the witness during the preliminary hearing and the witness was not available for cross-examination during trial made the witness' transcript inadmissible.

The US Supreme Court reversed the ruling by the Ohio Supreme Court. Justice Blackmun wrote the opinion of the Court and was joined by Justices Burger, Stewart, Powell, and Rehnquist. The Justices found that the original testimony by Anita met the "indicia of reliability" requirement and that Anita was unavailable for trial. Based on these two facts, the transcript of her testimony was admissible.

The dissent, written by Justice Brennan and joined by Justices Marshall and Stevens, argued that the State failed to meet the requirement of producing Anita for court. Sending five subpoenas to the residence of Anita's parents was not a "good-faith effort" to locate the witness. Justice Brennan opined that the State would have exerted a much greater effort to locate the witness if it didn't have her statement from the preliminary hearing.

*Ohio v. Roberts* set forth the standard that a statement is admissible if it is found to be reliable and trustworthy. If the statement is deemed sufficiently reliable, cross-examination is not necessary and the Confrontation Clause is not violated. This opinion set the precedent that an analytical report found to be trustworthy could be admitted without testimony, and likewise cross-examination, of the witness.

### 1.1.2 *Crawford v. Washington*, 541 U.S. 36 (2004). Argued November 10, 2003 – decided March 8, 2004

The opinion of *Ohio v. Roberts* was overturned by *Crawford v. Washington*. In this case the Court opined that cross-examination is the only way to satisfy the Confrontation Clause. The witness must be available to be questioned by the accused and the jury must be able to observe his response and measure his truthfulness. The facts of the case are given in the following.

Michael Crawford and his wife Sylvia entered the apartment of Kenneth Lee to confront him. Sylvia claimed that Kenneth had attempted to rape her. An altercation ensued and Michael stabbed Kenneth. Michael and Sylvia were arrested, received their Miranda warnings and were separately interrogated by detectives on two separate occasions. Both individuals gave ambiguous and similar statements regarding whether or not the victim wielded a weapon at the time of the stabbing. Sylvia did not testify during the trial. Washington has a state marital privilege which bars a spouse from testifying without the other spouse's consent. However, the court admitted Sylvia's statement under the standard set forth by *Ohio v. Roberts* reasoning that the out-of-court statement was sufficiently reliable based on the fact that the defendant and the witness gave similar statements independently on two occasions. The defense argued that admission of the statement without the opportunity for cross-examination violated the accused's right to confront the witness. The court found the statement admissible and the jury found the defendant guilty.

The Washington Court of Appeals reversed the decision. The court focused on the trustworthiness of Sylvia's out-of-court testimony and found it to be unreliable on several points: it contradicted one of her earlier statements; the statement was a response to a specific question; and, she admitted to closing her eyes during the altercation. On appeal, the Washington Supreme Court reinstated the conviction. The court agreed with the trial court's opinion that the statement of the defendant and the witness were nearly identical and therefore reliable.

The US Supreme Court reversed the decision on the grounds that Sylvia's statement was inadmissible. The Justices came to this decision through careful examination of the history of the Confrontation Clause, finding that it was not limited to in-court testimony. The spirit of the Sixth Amendment was to allow a witness to confront any accuser regardless of how the accusation was being introduced into the trial: out-of-court statement or in-court testimony. The Court's ruling and subsequent cases define a new standard that cross-examination was the only acceptable means of satisfying the Confrontation Clause for statements that are deemed to be testimonial (Garvey 2013). The following case defined "testimonial" in the eye of the Court.

### 1.1.3  *Melendez-Diaz v. Massachusetts*, 557 U.S. 305 (2009). Argued November 10, 2008 – decided June 25, 2009

Thomas Wright was a Kmart employee who was engaged in suspicious behavior. Wright regularly received a phone call during work after which he was picked up by a blue sedan in front of the store and then returned after a short time. The police were alerted to this suspicious activity by Wright's co-worker and set up surveillance in the Kmart parking lot. The police witnessed this activity and detained Wright when he returned from one of these short trips. They found four clear baggies containing a white powdery substance in Wright's possession. Additional police officers were called to the scene and they arrested two passengers in the car. The officers placed the three men in a police car and drove them to the police station. During the drive, the police witnessed one of the arrestees fidgeting in the back seat. Once they were back at the police station, the officer searched the car and found, hidden in the car seat, a baggie holding 19 smaller baggies each containing a white powdery substance.

Luis Melendez-Diaz was one of the three men arrested during the event and was charged with distributing and trafficking cocaine. The trial judge admitted into evidence the baggies of white powdery substance seized from Wright and the police car and three certificates of analysis. The certificates of analysis showed that the seized substance was found to contain cocaine. The certificates of analysis were sworn to before a notary public by analysts of the State Laboratory Institute of Massachusetts Department of Public Health.

Defense counsel objected to the admission of the certificates, stating that the US Supreme Court's decision in *Crawford v. Washington* required the analysts to testify in person. The objection was overruled and the certificates were admitted pursuant to state law that recognized the certificates as accurate until proven otherwise. The jury found Melendez-Diaz guilty.

Melendez-Diaz appealed on the grounds that the admission of the certificates violated the Confrontation Clause. The Appeals Court of Massachusetts rejected the claim and upheld the guilty verdict.

The US Supreme Court accepted review of the case. The majority decision saw the crux of the issue as whether a certificate of analysis was "testimonial," rendering the analyst who authored it a witness subject to the defendant's right of confrontation under the Sixth Amendment. The majority concluded that the certificates of analysis were affidavits created for the purpose of establishing or proving a fact, and accordingly were equivalent to live, in-person testimony. Further, the Justices stated that it was reasonable to assume that the analyst was aware of the evidentiary purpose of the certificate. In light of the *Crawford* decision, certificates of analysis were testimonial statements and analysts were witnesses for the purpose of the Sixth Amendment.

Four Justices dissented, arguing that the analyst was not an "accusatory" witness, and that the analyst's testimony was impactful only when considered with other evidence linking the defendant to the contraband. However, the majority clearly articulated that the Confrontation Clause of the Sixth Amendment speaks to two types of witnesses: witnesses against the defendant; and witnesses in his favor. There is no third type of witness, i.e. a witness that is advantageous to the prosecution, but immune to cross-examination.

The dissent further argued that the testimony provided at trial (certificate of analysis) is neutral, resulting from scientific testing. They suspected that the analyst would not alter the findings of his report when forced to confront his witness. The majority responded that the National Academy of Sciences report *Strengthening Forensic Science in the United States: A Path Forward* is contrary to this argument, in as much as it highlights the weaknesses of forensic science and identifies serious deficiencies that have been found in forensic evidence used in trial (Edwards 2010). The Justices recognized that an honest analyst will not change his testimony, but a fraudulent analyst may. Further, a poorly trained and deficient analyst may be disclosed during cross-examination. The Justices accordingly confirmed the right of confrontation as one means of assuring accurate forensic analysis, although not the ideal method to identify poor science.

Also, of importance was the quality of the certificate of analysis. The report solely identified the seized substance as containing cocaine. The report did not identify the method used to test the substance or indicate if the method was routine, nor did it state if the results involved interpretation, thereby increasing the potential for human error. These concerns additionally could have been explored during cross-examination.

Of interest, the dissent noted that the majority's decision referred to "an analyst," but failed to define that term. Therefore, an analyst could be anyone who played a role in the testing including analysts, technicians, and even the individual who calibrates the equipment. The dissent warned that this vagueness could put undue pressure on the forensic science community as prosecutors called and defense required a parade of witnesses.

### 1.1.4  *Bullcoming v. New Mexico*, 564 U.S. 647 (2011). Argued March 2, 2011 – decided June 23, 2011

In *Bullcoming v. New Mexico,* the Supreme Court was faced with evaluating the appropriateness of surrogate witnesses. Donald Bullcoming was arrested on charges of driving while intoxicated (DWI). During trial, the prosecution admitted the laboratory report certifying that Bullcoming's blood alcohol concentration was above the legal limit. The prosecution did not call the original analyst, who was on unpaid leave at the time of the trial, to testify; instead, they called an alternate analyst. The alternate analyst was certified and performed the same analyses following the same methods on a regular basis; however, he did not observe the original analyst perform the test or supervise his work.

The defense learned of the surrogate analyst during the trial and was caught by surprise. Bullcoming's counsel argued that admission of the laboratory report without an opportunity to cross-examine the original analyst was a violation of the defendant's Sixth Amendment right. The judge overruled the objection and admitted the analytical report as a business record. The court convicted Bullcoming on the charge of aggravated DWI.

The New Mexico Court of Appeals upheld the lower court ruling. The Court of Appeals concluded that the blood alcohol report was non-testimonial and routinely prepared. The nature of the documents ensured trustworthiness under the *Ohio v. Roberts* opinion.

While Bullcoming's case was pending appeal before the New Mexico Supreme Court, the US Supreme Court delivered its opinion in *Melendez-Diaz v. Massachusetts*. As previously stated, this opinion clearly identified analytical reports as testimony. In light of this ruling, the New Mexico Supreme Court recognized the analytical report as testimony, but still found it admissible. The Court reasoned that the original analyst was simply transferring information from a machine (gas chromatograph) to a report. And, although the surrogate analyst did not observe the original analyst at work or supervise his work, the surrogate analyst, being qualified to operate the gas chromatograph, could testify to the findings in the report. The Court acknowledged that it was imperative for an analyst to testify because neither the analytical machine nor the report could be questioned; however, the surrogate was sufficient to preserve the defendant's right to confrontation.

On appeal, the US Supreme Court rejected this reasoning, holding that the witness who made the out-of-court testimony (in this case signed the analytical report) must be available for cross-examination. The Justices found that there was much more involved in performing the analytical test than simply transferring data from an instrument to a report. For example, the analyst received the evidence in its original state, ensured the case number was correctly reported, and determined that the instrument was functioning correctly. The accused had the right to confront the analyst who actually handled the evidence and produced the certificate. A surrogate witness could not answer to what the original witness knew or observed about the events he certified, nor expose any of that analyst's deficiencies. Justice Ginsburg summarized the Court's opinion by stating, "we hold that surrogate testimony of that order does not meet the constitutional requirement" (*Bullcoming v. New Mexico* 2011, para. 4).

The dissenting Justices (Kennedy, Roberts, Alito, and Breyer) raised concerns regarding multistep forensic analysis that involved more than one analyst. They questioned how the court, prosecution, and defense would know which analyst or technician should be called to testify. Should every analyst and technician who was involved in the analysis be called?

### 1.1.5 *Williams v. Illinois*, 567 U.S. 50 (2012). Argued December 6, 2011 – decided June 18, 2012

In this case, the Justices made the muddy waters even murkier by failing to reach a majority decision. In *Williams v. Illinois*, a female was abducted, robbed, and raped by a stranger. The victim immediately reported the crime to the police and a rape kit was collected. The vaginal swabs were sent to a private laboratory for analysis. DNA profiles of the perpetrator were identified and uploaded into the state's DNA database. The computer system indicated a match with a DNA profile obtained from a sample of Sandy Williams. The victim later identified Sandy Williams as the perpetrator from a police lineup.

During trial, the prosecution called the analyst from the state laboratory that obtained Williams' DNA profile as well as the DNA analyst who compared the profile obtained at the private laboratory and the profile obtained at the state laboratory, but did not call the analyst from the private laboratory. The analyst who compared the DNA profiles testified that the private laboratory was accredited and the results reported by the laboratory were regularly relied upon, but did not elaborate on the procedures used by the private laboratory. The defense counsel argued that not being able to cross-examine the analyst who obtained the DNA profile from the vaginal swabs violated the defendant's right to confront the witness. The prosecutor countered that the defendant's rights were satisfied, because he had the opportunity to cross-examine the analyst who had matched the two DNA profiles, i.e. the analyst who had identified Mr. Williams as the perpetrator. The court admitted the evidence and found the defendant guilty. The Court of Appeals and State Supreme Court upheld the ruling.

Unfortunately, the US Supreme Court did not come to a majority opinion. Justices Alito, Kennedy, and Breyer concluded that the testimony did not violate the Confrontation Clause. Justice Thomas agreed, but based on different reasons. The plurality found that the question at hand was whether or not an analyst could speak to a testimonial statement (i.e. analytical report) of another analyst if that report was not being admitted as evidence. The Justices felt that based on the circumstantial evidence (identifying the perpetrator from the police lineup) and the documented chain of custody, the DNA profile obtained by the private laboratory was what it purported to be. Furthermore, if the prosecution had questioned the analyst using the traditionally accepted practice of hypothetical questioning, there would be no concerns in regards to the Confrontation Clause. The Justices also concluded that the private laboratory report was not testimonial, because it did not identify a particular suspect and that the results could not be skewed to identify a particular suspect.

Justice Thomas agreed that the testimony did not violate the Confrontation Clause, but based on a different reason. Justice Thomas felt that the private laboratory's report was not testimonial. The report was not certified nor was it sworn to; therefore, it was not a testimonial statement.

Justice Kagan filed the dissenting opinion and was joined by Justices Scalia, Ginsburg, and Sotomayor. All four Justices saw no difference between this case and *Bullcoming* or *Melendez-Diaz*. They felt the private laboratory's report was offered for its truth and was out-of-court testimony; therefore, it was subject to the Confrontation Clause. They disagreed with the plurality opinion that a statement had to be directed at an individual to be recognized as testimonial. Also, they rejected Justice Thomas' rational for admitting the uncertified laboratory report, noting that the formality requirement was rejected by the Court in *Bullcoming* (Garvey 2013).

## 1.2   Impact on forensic practitioners

Each US Supreme Court decision presented here is a direct response to a specific case issue that has repercussions on the general practice of forensic science without clear direction. The decisions do not provide judges, prosecutors, and defendants with defined pathways for handling complex forensic analyses and allow for a large amount of interpretation (see Appendix). Conservative prosecutors may choose to produce every technician or analyst who was involved in forensic testing at any level for court testimony (Garvey 2013). This creates a great burden on forensic laboratories. The laboratory management and employees should have an understanding of these US Supreme Court decisions and prepare the laboratory staff to respond appropriately.

The Court's opinion in *Melendez-Diaz* clarified that the analytical report is out-of-court testimony and the analyst is subject to the Confrontation Clause. However, it failed to define the analyst, leaving all individuals who handle evidence a potential witness. *Williams v. Illinois* further failed to clarify who should be called to testify when forensic analyses involve multiple individuals.

Justice Kagan notes that calling the "lead" analyst to testify should be adequate, but she is not writing for the plurality opinion and this note carries very little weight (*Williams v. Illinois*). The failure to define the analyst potentially puts untrained individuals on the stand jeopardizing the laboratory's reputation and the bearing of the analytical findings on the trial. In response, laboratories must clearly define the role of each employee involved in handling evidence and prepare each for court testimony. Consider a student working in a Forensic Anthropology laboratory. The student may be trained and assigned to the role of receiving, inventorying, and accessioning skeletal evidence. However, in the learning environment of the laboratory, the student observes the development of the biological profile and attends pretrial meetings.

By the time of trial, the student has greater visibility of the case than simply the receiving, inventory, and accessioning of skeletal evidence. However, during testimony, the student must speak only to his or her role in the case and not to the analysis or conclusions. The student must be prepared to direct the questioner to the correct person when questioned about components of the analysis outside his or her defined role.

Learning to limit responses to information which is solely within an individual's expertise is difficult, especially when the individual has much greater knowledge of the case in its entirety; however, it is essential to prevent the individual from speaking to elements of the case about which he/she is not trained nor qualified as an expert. Strong standard operating procedures and clearly written position descriptions are the laboratory's best defense for preparing for the impact of *Melendez-Diaz*.

Despite the right to a speedy trial as dictated by the Sixth Amendment, the period between analysis of evidence and court testimony can be years. This lengthy interval creates a real need for surrogate witnesses; however, the *Bullcoming* decision severely limits the use of surrogate witnesses (*Bullcoming v. New Mexico*). Essentially, the ruling dictates that an analyst cannot testify to another analyst's report; each analyst must reach a conclusion based on independent analysis.

This ruling directly impacts laboratory practices in two ways. First, adequate samples must be collected to allow for additional testing and these samples must be archived, when possible. In the written decision, the Justices recognized that an archived sample is often available for additional testing and advocate for retesting rather than use of a surrogate witness (*Bullcoming v. New Mexico*). The Court decisions do not provide guidance on required retention schedules of these samples; although, some state laws do. Secondly, when a sample cannot be archived or the analytical process is destructive (e.g. performing an autopsy, excavating a grave), the analysis must be sufficiently documented to enable an alternate analyst to form an opinion based on independent observation of the data.

The role of Forensic Anthropology in medico-legal investigations is growing. More medical examiner offices are employing in-house anthropologists or consulting university-based anthropologists. As employment opportunities increase so does the movement of practitioners between these jobs. The transiency of practitioners along with retirement, injury, and death makes the need for surrogate testimony a reality. Furthermore, skeletal remains are often not available by the time a case is adjudicated. When the original analyst and the skeletal remains are unavailable, a second analyst must work from photographs, diagrams, and raw data to form an independent opinion. Depending on the attorney, the analyst may or may not have access to the original report. Therefore, the original analyst must document a case in a manner that allows another practitioner to form an independent opinion.

The original anthropologist must document and photograph each feature used to build the biological profile. The same holds for each traumatic finding and abnormality. All measurements must be clearly recorded. Any metric analyses must be retained as part of the case record. Documentation of negative findings should be considered as well. A unique case identifier must be clearly listed on each item in order to maintain chain of custody. These items must be archived in a way that ensures their availability for the foreseeable future. Poor record keeping can jeopardize the admissibility of the analysis. Chapters 6 and 7 in this volume provide extensive guidance for case report documentation.

The presented US Supreme Court decisions place a burden on forensic laboratories, but in many ways strengthen them. They guide laboratory management to develop well defined position descriptions and standard operating procedures. They underscore the need for adequate analyst training. They promote adequate record keeping. As the intersection between forensic science and the law broadens, forensic scientists must keep abreast of the impact of Supreme Court decisions.

## 1.A  Appendix

### Case study – confrontation clause

A forensic pathologist moved jurisdiction from Florida to Arizona. After being employed in the new office for several months she received a request to testify in a capital murder trial in Florida. Initially she cited the case load at her new office and declined the request. The prosecutor's office issued a subpoena. Subpoenas are valid only for the jurisdiction in which they are served, therefore she was not compelled to respond. However she did begin discussions with her new Chief and the office attorney and they also cited the burden to the office in their refusal. The prosecutor in Florida filed an "Application for Certificate Compelling Witness to Appear" in the Superior Court in Arizona. The Arizona Judge granted the certificate and the pathologist was compelled to appear in Florida. The Florida Judge issued some fairly harsh criticism of the pathologist (see below).

Judge's Comments:

> "We're not going to have a situation where a person who's having his life on the line … is going to have the case jeopardized because of game playing," the judge said. He ordered [her] to prepare and to testify or face "direct criminal contempt."

> [The Judge] noted that it's often hard to get witnesses with rap sheets "a mile long" to testify truthfully in criminal cases, and then remarked on "how absolutely amazing it is that we have a professional who is a medical examiner whose duty is to do justice … who refuses to review the materials and wants to play games."

> [Pathologist], who now has a similar position in Arizona, initially said she could not provide complete testimony until a formal agreement was worked out between her former employer and her current one.

> *(Krueger 2015)*

Since that time, two other pathologists from that office have been subpoenaed back to their previous jurisdictions and in both cases the Arizona Judge has upheld the subpoena. The Judge's comments in this case may appear to be unfair given that the pathologist refused to testify because of a wrangle between her current office, the previous office, and the State's Attorney. However, it gives insight into the type of pressure and exposure that experts face due to the confrontation clause and the subsequent confusion created by the legal rulings about it.

## 1.A.1  Example of Florida application to compel testimony

---

**Application:**

IN THE CIRCUIT COURT OF THE SIXTH JUDICIAL CIRCUIT OF THE STATE OF FLORIDA

[Case number redacted]

STATE OF FLORIDA

v                                                    MURDER IN THE FIRST DEGREE

Defendant

APPLICATION FOR CERTIFICATE COMPELLING ATTENDANCE OF WITNESS

Comes now, [prosecutor name] State Attorney for the Sixth Judicial Circuit of Florida, and moves this Honorable Court to grant this Application for Certificate Compelling Attendance of Witness, pursuant to Florida Statute 942.03, and bases the said application on the following:

1. [Pathologist], M.D. is a material and necessary witness for the State of Florida in prosecution of the above criminal case now pending before this Court... [Redacted].

2. Trial in the above case is currently set on... [Redacted] at the [Redacted]. This Court has jurisdiction to try this felony case in...[Redacted].

3. The presence of [pathologist] will be required on [Redacted] at the Office of the State Attorney, for the entire day beginning at 8:30 a.m. at the [Redacted] County Justice Center [Redacted], Florida to give testimony for the State of Florida in this criminal case.

---

## 1.A.2 Example of Arizona court order in response to Florida request

WILLIAM G. MONTGOMERY
MARICOPA COUNTY ATTORNEY

IN THE SUPERIOR COURT OF THE STATE OF ARIZONA IN AND FOR THE COUNTY OF MARICOPA

THE STATE OF ARIZONA,
IN THE MATTER OF THE
APPLICATION OF THE STATE
OF FLORIDA FOR AN ORDER
REQUIRING ONE
   [PATHOLOGIST]
TO APPEAR AS WITNESS BEFORE       ORDER DIRECTING WITNESS
THE SIXTH JUDICIAL CIRCUIT COURT     TO APPEAR AND TESTIFY
OF THE STATE OF FLORIDA,                IN [REDACTED] COUNTY,
COUNTY OF [REDACTED]                  FLORIDA

Whereas, IT APPEARING to the satisfaction of this court that [PATHOLOGIST] is a necessary and material witness for the State of Florida, in Case No. [Redacted], entitled *State of Florida v* [Redacted].

NOW THEREFORE IT IS HEREBY ORDERED AND DIRECTED that the said [Pathologist] appear before the Sixth Judicial Circuit Court of the State of Florida, in and for the County of [Redacted], located in the [Redacted] County Justice Center, [address redacted], on or about the [Redacted] as witness for the State of Florida in the above stated cause.

FURTHERMORE, failure without good cause to appear as directed may subject the said witness to citation for contempt of court and, if convicted, imprisonment and/or fine.

DATED this _____ day of _____, _____

_____signature redacted_____
Judge of the Superior Court of the
State of Arizona, in and for the County
Of Maricopa

# References

Bibas S, & Fisher JL. (n.d.). Common interpretation: The Sixth Amendment. https://constitutioncenter.org/interactive-constitution/amendments/amendment-vi (accessed May 29, 2018).

*Bullcoming v. New Mexico,* 564 U.S. 647 (2011). Justia. https://supreme.justia.com/cases/federal/us/564/647 (accessed June 6, 2018).

*Crawford v. Washington,* 541 U.S. 36 (2004). FindLaw. https://caselaw.findlaw.com/us-supreme-court/541/36.html (accessed May 29, 2018).

Edwards, H.T. (2010). *The National Academy of Sciences report on forensic sciences: What it means for the bench and bar*. District of Columbia.

Garvey, T.M. (2013). *Williams v. Illinois* and forensic evidence: the bleeding edge of *Crawford*. *Strategies: The Prosecutor's. Newsletter on Violence Against Women* 11: 1–11.

Krueger, C. (2015). Pinellas man facing death penalty in killing of two year old girl. *Tampa Bay Times* (January 21). www.tampabay.com (accessed June 19, 2018).

*Melendez-Diaz v. Massachusetts*, 557 U.S. 305 (2009). FindLaw. https://caselaw.findlaw.com/us-supreme-court/557/305.html (accessed May 29, 2018).

*Ohio v. Roberts*, 448 U.S. 56 (1980). FindLaw. https://caselaw.findlaw.com/us-supreme-court/448/56.html (accessed May 29, 2018).

*Williams v. Illinois*, 567 U.S. 50 (2012). FindLaw. https://caselaw.findlaw.com/us-supreme-court/10-8505.html (accessed May 29, 2018).

# CHAPTER 2

# "Somewhere in this twilight": the circumstances leading to the National Academy of Sciences' report

Thomas Holland[1] and Christian Crowder[2]

[1] United States Department of Defense, POW/MIA Accounting Agency, Washington, DC, USA
[2] Southwestern Institute of Forensic Sciences, Dallas, TX, USA

## 2.1 Introduction

In 1993, the Supreme Court fired a shot across the bow of the forensic science world when it issued its majority opinion in the landmark *Daubert v. Merrell Dow* (1993) case. On its face, the Court did little more than affirm the supremacy of the Federal Rules of Evidence (FRE) for use in federal courts. Viewed in a more nuanced framework, however, the seven justices who comprised the majority behind the opinion appeared to send a clear and unequivocal message to the lower courts: do a better job of judicial "gatekeeping."

The message was received, and federal courts soon saw a ratcheting up of the scrutiny given scientific expert testimony, particularly as it related to reliability of the evidence. A 2001 study by the Rand Institute for Civil Justice (Dixon and Gill 2001) concluded that in the years immediately following the Supreme Court's 1993 *Daubert* ruling, the number of successful challenges to experts' qualifications and evidence reliability rose. The authors of the Rand Study attribute this trend to judges "doing what they were directed to do by the Supreme Court: increasingly acting as gatekeepers for reliability and relevance" (Dixon and Gill 2001, p. 64).

But the *Daubert* case did not arise in a vacuum. It is true that the different federal circuits had not shown complete uniformity in their applications of the FRE following its promulgation in 1975, but these differing applications had not yet diverged to a point where the equitable administration of justice was endangered. Why then did *Daubert* come about? And how did it lead, 16 years later, to the National Academy of Sciences' (NAS) report that found

*Forensic Anthropology and the United States Judicial System*, First Edition.
Edited by Laura C. Fulginiti, Kristen Hartnett-McCann, and Alison Galloway.
© 2019 John Wiley & Sons Ltd. Published 2019 by John Wiley & Sons Ltd.

the state of forensic science in the United States to be "seriously wanting"? (National Research Council 2009, p. 13). The answer lies partly in what else was happening in the United States in the realm of civil law in the 1970s and 1980s and how the admissibility of expert evidence had evolved over those years. And to understand that, one must begin somewhere in the twilight.

This chapter traces the evolving evidentiary standards in US courts from the early days of scientific testimony in the courtroom, through the toxic tort litigation of the late nineteenth century, up to the modern *Daubert* standard and its progeny.

## 2.2   The long road to *Daubert*

### 2.2.1   The *Frye* standard of general acceptance

On the evening of November 27, 1920, Robert W. Brown, a prominent Black physician and business man was shot to death in the hallway of his home in Washington, DC (Slain in Home 1920). Despite the presence of an eyewitness to the shooting, and the fact that the murder garnered newspaper coverage across the country, the DC police were unable to develop any likely suspects, and as time went on, the trail grew increasingly cold. Then, almost nine months later, the police caught an unlikely break; James Alphonso Frye, a 26-year-old Black male in jail on an unrelated robbery charge, confessed to the Brown shooting, and moreover, he did so in enough detail (Confesses to Murder 1921) that it left little doubt in the minds of the police as to his guilt. The story might have easily ended there, with James Frye just another name on a forgotten court record, were it not for the fact that shortly before the trial began, he completely recanted his story, claiming that he had been tricked into confessing by the police and that he had no involvement in the murder.

Frye's flip-flop presented his two relatively inexperienced lawyers with a simple, yet substantial, dilemma: their client had now made two statements – the 1921 detailed confession and the subsequent 1922 recantation – only one of which could be true. As the trial began on July 17, 1922, the defense team struggled with the problem of how to best convince the jury that James Frye was being truthful when he recanted his earlier confession and was lying when he originally talked to the police (Lepore 2015a). As fate would have it, in the months immediately before the trial began, Frye's two defense lawyers had enrolled in a first-of-a-kind course at American University in Washington, DC, entitled *Legal Psychology*, which was taught by the attorney and noted psychologist, William Moulton Marston (Lepore 2015a). Professor Marston had for years researched the accuracy and underlying psychology of eyewitness accounts, but by the time of Frye's trial, Marston's interest had shifted to demonstrating the physiological response associated with lying. Marston was convinced that he could use changes in an individual's systolic blood pressure to ferret out deceptive statements, i.e. the *Lie Detector*, and when Marston learned of Frye's predicament, he jumped at the opportunity to assist his former students and to prove his theory in court. With Frye's acquiescence, Professor Marston administered his "systolic blood pressure deception test" – a forerunner of the modern polygraph – to Frye in the DC jail and, to the defense team's delight, Marston concluded that Frye's 1922 recantation that he had no involvement in Dr. Brown's murder was in fact the truthful statement (Lepore 2015a).

But having an opinion is one thing, and getting that opinion in front of a jury proved to be another matter altogether. On July 20, Frye's lawyers attempted to offer Professor Marston's expert testimony into evidence only to encounter a judge with no desire to depart from judicial norms and even less patience for novel and unproven science. "[I]t is for the jury to determine whether or not [Frye] was telling the truth," when he recanted his confession, Judge Walter McCoy told the lawyers in denying their attempt (Lepore 2015a, p. 1128) and "I have gotten too old and too much inured to certain general principles in regard to the trial of cases to depart from them rashly" (Lepore 2015a, p. 1134). Marston's opinion was not introduced, and the jury, after deliberating less than an hour, convicted James Frye of second-degree murder, largely on the basis of his initial confession (Starrs 1982).[1]

The story may have ended with Frye's incarceration except for the fact that his lawyers appealed his conviction and thus set into motion one of the landmark decisions by a US appellate court. On appeal for error, Frye's lawyers argued, inter alia (among other things), that Marston's revolutionary testimony had been improperly withheld from the jury, and as a result, Frye's right to a fair trial had been violated. On December 3, 1923, in a markedly terse 665-word opinion, Associate Justice Josiah Van Orsdel of the Court of Appeals of the District of Columbia made short work of the defense argument, affirming the trial court's verdict and in the process, articulating what would become known as the *Frye* standard for the admission of scientific evidence.

> Just when a scientific principle or discovery crosses the line between the experimental and demonstrable stages is difficult to define. Somewhere in this twilight zone the evidential force of the principle must be recognized, and while courts will go a long way in admitting expert testimony deduced from a well-recognized scientific principle or discovery, the thing from which the deduction is made must be sufficiently established to have gained general acceptance in the particular field in which it belongs.
>
> *(Frye 1923, p. 1014).*

Running headlong into a conservative judge was Frye's misfortune, but it also did not help that while his case was going up on appeal, Marston was arrested and arraigned on charges of fraud stemming from an unrelated business venture

(Lepore 2015a). Ultimately, the charges against Marston were dropped, but not until a full month after Justice Van Orsdel had penned his laconic opinion in *Frye* that may have forever doomed the admissibility of the polygraph. To what extent Professor Marston's ill-fated business dealings played in Frye's future is not clear, but certainly the key expert witness being charged with fraud likely did not favorably incline the judges in Frye's direction. Reading the rather clear writing on the wall, James Frye's lawyers never filed an appeal to the US Supreme Court, and Frye spent the next sixteen years in federal penitentiaries, before receiving parole in June 1939.

For his part, William Marston left American University and began teaching at Tufts University in Boston, but his story was far from over. While there, he became romantically involved with one of his graduate students, who ultimately moved in with the Professor and his wife, and the three of them lived together for the remainder of their lives, with Marston fathering children with both women (Lepore 2015b). His academic career effectively ended, William Moulton Marston headed for Hollywood where he worked as a story advisor for Universal Studios, conducting psychological studies of target audiences – known as focus groups today (Lepore 2015b). There, in Hollywood, Professor Marston got his final word on lie detection. Writing under the pen-name, Charles Moulton, he created the character of Wonder Woman, and, perhaps not surprisingly, given his history and his marital situation, he equipped his superhero with the ultimate lie detector – a Golden Lasso of Truth, the efficacy of which was not left up to the general acceptance of the scientific community or the inurement of an elderly federal judge.

What would have been the outcome had Marston been allowed to testify? Had he not been indicted for fraud, and had he not embarked upon a scandalous marital arrangement that effectively derailed his on-going research, would the polygraph be admissible today? No one knows, but what is known is that the *Frye* standard, or "General Acceptance" test, soon was adopted by the other Federal circuits and became the de facto standard for a majority of both federal and state courts evaluating the admissibility of scientific expert testimony (Giannelli 1994). The central question of whether or not a scientific principle was generally accepted by the relevant community was to remain the seminal benchmark test for the next seventy years.

## 2.3   The federal rules of evidence

Beginning in the mid-1960s, the US Supreme Court undertook an extensive review of the existing standards for the admissibility of evidence in federal courts and the need for greater uniformity. The Court had overseen the drafting of the Federal Rules of Civil Procedure in 1938, with great success, and it was determined that the procedures for handling evidence would similarly benefit. The result was the promulgation of the FRE, which were signed into law on January 2, 1975,[2] and immediately became applicable in all federal courts.

Rule 702, as adopted in 1975, provided:

> If scientific, technical, or other specialized knowledge will assist the trier of fact to understand the evidence or to determine a fact in issue, a witness qualified as an expert by knowledge, skill, experience, training, or education, may testify thereto in the form of an opinion or otherwise.
>
> (Fed. R. Evid. 702 (1975)).

Notably, and for unknown reasons, the drafters of the FRE did not adopt *Frye's General Acceptance* language when crafting the standard for expert testimony. Instead, Rule 702 as originally adopted focused on two essential prongs of expert testimony – its *relevance* to the matter at hand and the *overall quality* of the science and the qualifications of the individual scientist.

Federal courts immediately began applying the FRE to the admissibility of expert testimony, as was required by the law, but almost as quickly began encountering a problem. The emphasis on the relevance of the proffered testimony, i.e. the value of the testimony in helping the jury understand the evidence, was straightforward, but what proved problematic is that the FRE provided no guidance – as the *Frye* standard had provided – on how judges were to evaluate the *quality* of the science involved (Becker and Orenstein 1992). In federal courts, judges are given great leeway in deciding matters of evidence admissibility and are guided primarily by the doctrine of *stare decisis*, i.e. "to stand on that decided." Under this principle, judges follow precedential holdings from similar cases; however, only those cases decided by a higher court in the trial court's judicial hierarchy are binding. In the United States court system, federal trial courts are organized into districts, and districts are grouped into circuits (of which there currently are 12). In the absence of a Supreme Court ruling on a particular matter, the individual circuits are largely independent of one another. As a result, interpretations of law at the appellate circuit level, typically in appellate decisions, are binding on all lower federal district courts within that circuit – but are not binding on courts outside the circuit (though they may carry persuasive value). Consequently, as courts within the various circuits apply the law, subtle, and at times not so subtle, differences in interpretation develop among the circuits. Sometimes these differences can evolve to be so great as to jeopardize the equitable administration of justice. When that happens, the US Supreme Court typically steps in to resolve the confusion and its interpretation of the law becomes binding on all lower federal courts. This is the situation involving expert witnesses that began to slowly evolve following the promulgation of Rule 702.

## 2.4   The rise of the toxic tort

The 1980s saw the rise of what came to be called "toxic tort" litigation.[3] Through-out the late 1970s, but particularly during the 1980s, American courts were flooded with individual and class-action civil suits alleging injury from expo-sure to a variety of products such as asbestos, Agent Orange, the Dalkon Shield IUD, nuclear fallout, and a host of groundwater contaminates.[4] As different as these toxic tort cases sometimes were, they all had one thing in common; aside from the sometimes staggering monetary claims, each plaintiff was faced with the requirement of establishing a causative link between the agent and the injury. In almost all of these cases, establishing or severing the causal nexus was achieved through the testimony of scientists, medical professionals, and engineers on both sides of the claims. What also threads through these cases is the frequent inability of the courts to adequately deal with the admissibility of the expert testimony, a fact that arguably gave birth in the 1970s and 1980s to what became known as the era of "junk science." The "mix of opportunity and incentive," science writer Peter Huber argues, led to a legal environment where "almost any self-styled scientist, no matter how strange or iconoclastic his views, [was] welcome[d] to testify in court" (Huber 1993), and in perhaps no area of toxic tort litigation was this better illustrated than the rise of silicone breast implant cases.

Silicone was an unlikely villain. It was one of the wonder substances that helped the Allies win World War II; it is versatile, durable, and dependable, and it quickly found its way into a wide variety of products from airplane gaskets to nuclear submarine lubricants. Moreover, test after test had also shown it to be safe when injected into or ingested by humans, and it was just a matter of time before it found its way into the realm of surgical implants, both therapeutic and cosmetic.

In 1962, Timmie Jean Lindsey became the first woman to receive silicone breast implants, and by all accounts at the time, the procedure proved highly successful (Fisher 2015). The popularity of silicone-gel implants grew rapidly, and not surprisingly, the growth was accompanied by the occasional product lia-bility suit. Dow Corning, the largest manufacturer of silicone implants, quickly adopted a no-settlement posture, and it successfully weathered all such early claims until 1977, when a Cleveland woman successfully sued Dow Corning for injuries allegedly caused by silicone leakage from an implant (*V. Mueller & Co. v. Corley* 1978). Though the $170 000 settlement amount was modest by later stan-dards, the case signaled the beginning of a litigation feeding frenzy, and by early 1992, the FDA had forced silicone implants from the market, and by 1995, over 20 000 liability claims had driven Dow Corning to file Chapter 11 bankruptcy (Frontline, WGBH Educational Foundation n.d.).[5]

Dow Corning's problems likely seemed all too familiar to companies such as Johns-Manville and A.H. Robbins,[6] the companies behind asbestos and the Dalkon Shield IUD, but unlike their products, no credible evidence existed at the time to suggest that silicone implants posed a demonstrable health risk. Quite the contrary, study after study had shown no appreciable health risk, a conclusion that finally and conclusively was affirmed in 1999 by the Institute of Medicine (Institute of Medicine (US) Committee on the Safety of Silicone Breast Implants 1999).

If silicone is safe, why was Dow Corning[7] forced into nine years of Chapter 11 bankruptcy? The answer lies largely with the tendency of juries to exhibit "Hindsight Bias," that is, when confronted with "complicated and often contradictory scientific evidence in a typical personal injury or mass tort lawsuit, jurors will tend to reason back from what actually happened – viewing the evidence retrospectively – in order to determine what the defendant's prospective, pre-outcome conduct should have been" (Studebaker and Goodman-Delahunty 2002, p. 157).[8] But Hindsight Bias does not completely explain the rise of toxic torts seen in the 1970s and 1980s. Also playing a major role was the adoption by federal courts in 1975 of FRE 702 and its emphasis on relevancy. Juries only see what is presented to them, and the consequence of Rule 702 was that judges were now being asked to determine the relevancy of expert testimony without having the familiar backstop of *Frye*'s General Acceptance standard. For many largely science-illiterate judges, if an expert looked like a duck, and quacked like a duck, he or she should be able to testify as a duck. One scientist soon came to equal another, and as one appellate court characterized it, many judges adopted a "'let it all in' philosophy," that placed the onus on the jury to sort the wheat from the chaff (In re Air Crash Disaster 1986). This winnowing can be a daunting enough task if the sides are playing fairly, but in the era of toxic torts, where liability awards routinely were in the tens or hundreds of millions of dollars, self-proclaimed experts willing to shape facts to meet desired ends became all too common. "Junk science, to put things bluntly, [became] a very profitable business" (Huber 1993, p. 187).

It was into this evidentiary free-for-all that the Supreme Court stepped in 1993.

## 2.5  *Daubert* and the supremacy of the FRE

The members of the US Supreme Court may have been aware of the problems that the lower courts were struggling with, but they lacked the authority to do anything about it until someone brought them the issue in the form of a case. Unlike many state supreme courts, which can issue advisory opinions, the *Case or Controversy Clause* of the US Constitution requires that the US Supreme Court only adjudicate issues that have been brought before it as a legal case. So despite the turmoil roiling the lower courts, the Justices were required to wait until a case came in front of it; in 1993 that case was named *Daubert*.

The *Daubert*[9] case was actually a joining of two separate, but similar, cases. Jason Daubert and Eric Schuller were unrelated minor children who had been born with limb-reduction birth defects, caused, they argued, by their mothers taking the prescription anti-nausea drug, Bendectin, during the early stages of their pregnancies.

Bendectin was first approved by the FDA in 1956 for the treatment of nausea and vomiting in pregnancy, i.e. morning sickness. The formulation of the drug was refined through time and by 1976, it consisted of two common active ingredients, doxyamine succinate (an antihistamine commonly used as a sleep aid) and pyridoxine hydrochloride (Vitamin $B_6$) (Duchesnay Inc. 2017). In this formulation, Bendectin became the leading treatment for morning sickness in the United States and many other parts of the world. Yet, despite numerous studies that established the safety of Bendectin, Merrell Dow, the drug's manufacturer, was soon besieged with a series of product liability lawsuits alleging an association between the medication's use by pregnant women and an increased risk of birth defects. As had been the case with silicone breast implants, the rising cost of litigation ultimately made the product unprofitable, and in 1983, Merrell Dow pulled Bendectin from the market.[10] Nevertheless, the lawsuits continued through the 1980s and included those brought in federal court[11] by the guardians of Jason Daubert and Eric Schuller in 1989.

At trial, Daubert and Schuller attempted to introduce expert opinion evidence that an epidemiological reanalysis of *in vitro* and *in vivo* animal tests established a clear causal relationship between the active ingredients in Bendectin and limb-reduction birth defects (Daubert 1989). Dow Pharmaceuticals countered the argument by pointing out that no *published* epidemiological studies showed any statistically significant relationship between limb reductions and the drug and that a *reanalysis* of the data did not constitute a published epidemiological study. The trial judge, faced with the task of evaluating the quality of the science being proffered – as required by the FRE – turned to the tried-and-true *Frye* standard of general acceptance, and under that test found that the absence of published peer-reviewed studies strongly argued against the general acceptance of the plaintiffs' expert opinion. Accordingly, the trial judge ruled that Daubert's argument failed to meet its evidentiary burden, and he granted a motion for summary judgment, dismissing the case (Daubert 1989).

In April 1991, Daubert and Schuller filed for appeal with the Ninth Circuit Court of Appeals, but fared no better than they had at the trial court level. The FRE notwithstanding, the Ninth Circuit judges also adhered to a general-acceptance standard to evaluate quality of the evidence proffered by the *Daubert* lawyers and, as had the trial judge, found it wanting. "For expert opinion based on a given scientific methodology to be admissible, the methodology cannot diverge significantly from the procedures accepted by recognized authorities in the field," the court wrote. The judges found that although *Daubert's* experts had reanalyzed the epidemiological studies related to Bendectin's effects, the reanalysis did not "comply with this standard [in that] they were unpublished, not subjected to the normal peer review process, and [were] generated solely for use in litigation" (Daubert 1991, p. 1131). Accordingly, the court affirmed the trial judge's dismissal of the complaint and set the stage for the Supreme Court's review.

The Supreme Court heard arguments in *Daubert* on March 30, 1993, and issued its opinion 90 days later, vacating the lower court's ruling. Noting that the purpose of the FRE was to achieve a "relaxing [of] the traditional barriers to 'opinion testimony'," (Daubert 1993, p. 588) the 7–2 majority found that the "austere [*Frye*] standard, absent from, and incompatible with, the FRE, should not be applied in federal trials" (Daubert 1993, p. 589). The Court went on to emphasize "a gatekeeping role for the judge" of "ensuring that an expert's testimony both rests on a reliable foundation and is relevant to the task at hand" (Daubert 1993, p. 597).

But the problem that led to the Court's hearing of *Daubert* was less about the supremacy of the FRE and more about the lack of guidance on how to interpret and apply the FRE. Had the Supreme Court stopped with the holding that "the Frye test was superseded by the adoption of the Federal Rules of Evidence," (Daubert 1993, p. 587) it would have accomplished little. Fortunately, the Court, in rather detailed *obiter dicta* (by the way), provided a menu of "general observations" (Daubert 1993, p. 593) to assist trial judges in their role of gatekeeper.[12] Specifically, in what has come to be known as the *Daubert* standard, the Court stated that the judge should determine whether the scientific theory or technique (i) has been tested or can be tested, (ii) been published or subjected to peer review by the scientific community, (iii) has a known error rate or potential error rate, and (iv) enjoys widespread or general acceptance within the relevant scientific community (Daubert 1993, pp. 593–594).

Four years after *Daubert*, the Court again had an opportunity to address the issue of expert testimony when it decided *General Electric v. Joiner* (1997). Robert Joiner was an electrician who developed small-cell lung cancer, which he attributed to exposure to polychlorinated biphenyls (PCBs) used in electrical transformers. At trial the judge ruled that the opinion of Joiner's experts failed to establish a link between PCBs and lung cancer, and the case was dismissed in summary judgment. Joiner appealed to the Eleventh Circuit and won, and the defendant, General Electric, then took appeal to the Supreme Court. In affirming the trial court's decision, the Court ruled that it was within the trial judge's discretion to examine the soundness of an expert's conclusions. Thus, methodology and conclusions are not completely distinct from each other as had been suggested in *Daubert* (Godden and Walton 2006), and both should be examined by the judge (*Kumho Tire Co. v. Carmichael* 1999).[13]

Following *Daubert v. Merrell Dow Pharmaceuticals, Inc., General Electric Co. v. Joiner,* and *Kumho Tire Co. v. Carmichael* (see Glossary) (often referred to as the *Daubert* trilogy), pressure was mounting to resolve the conflicts in the courts regarding the meaning and interpretation of *Daubert*. In 2000, the following amendment was approved in order to provide more guidance on how to interpret and apply the FRE.

A witness who is qualified as an expert by knowledge, skill, experience, training, or education may testify in the form of an opinion or otherwise if:

(a)  The expert's scientific, technical, or other specialized knowledge will help the trier of fact to understand the evidence or to determine a fact in issue.
(b)  The testimony is based on sufficient facts or data.
(c)  The testimony is the product of reliable principles and methods.
(d)  The expert has reliably applied the principles and methods to the facts of the case.

   (As amended April 17, 2000, United States 1975, Rule 702).

## 2.6   The aftermath of *Daubert*

The 2001 Rand Study (Dixon and Gill 2001) suggests that in the wake of the *Daubert* decision, lower courts did in fact narrow the standards applied to expert testimony; however, at least one legal scholar argues that any tightening of the evidentiary sieve was merely temporary and that by 1997 the overall percentage of expert evidence ruled inadmissible had more-or-less returned to where it had been in the latter half of the 1980s (Billauer 2016). That is not to say, however, that the nature of the challenges remained the same through time.

Because *Daubert* hearings generally revolve around the qualifications of a proffered expert, it is easy to forget that the intended focus is less on the individual and more on the quality of the science that underlays the intended testimony. Whether it was the Court's intent or not, *Daubert* effectively opened a door, and what came tumbling out surprised everyone.

## 2.7   Llera Plaza and the assault on fingerprints

Fingerprinting is the grandfather of forensic science. Friction-ridge analysis has been used in US courts for over one hundred years – largely without serious question. In 1911, the Illinois Supreme Court became the first state supreme court to affirm that "the classification of finger-print impressions and their method of identification is a science requiring study" (*People v. Jennings* 1911, p. 1083). The court also took the opportunity to address the nature of expert testimony. In language that presaged *Daubert*, the court wrote that "[e]xpert testimony" such as that of a fingerprint examiner "is admissible when the subject matter of the inquiry is of such a character that only persons of skill and experience in it are capable of forming a correct judgment as to any facts connected therewith" (*People v. Jennings* 1911, p. 1082).

Such was the state of friction-ridge analysis on January 7, 2002, when federal judge Louis Pollak rendered his post-*Daubert* opinion in favor of Carlos Llera Plaza's motion to preclude the government from introducing latent fingerprint evidence in his murder trial.[14] In Judge Pollak's opinion (sometimes referred to as Plaza I) fingerprinting, as practiced in the United States, failed to meet the first three *Daubert* factors: it has not been "scientifically" tested, has not been "scientifically" peer reviewed, does not conform to uniform "scientific" standards, and may or may not be able to demonstrate a "scientific" rate of error. Science, Science, Science. Ironically, in the judge's opinion only *Daubert's* fourth factor, general acceptance by the relevant professional community – the old *Frye* standard – appeared to have been met (*United States v. Plaza* 2002, p. 552).

Predictably, given the volume of cases that had been grounded on fingerprint evidence, the government quickly moved for reconsideration of Judge Pollak's ruling on the grounds that the court's decision was "factually and legally flawed" (*United States v. Plaza* 2002, p. 553). On March 13, 2002, the judge reversed himself, vacating his January exclusionary order, and writing "[i]n short, I have changed my mind" (*United States v. Plaza* 2002, p. 576).

In reaching his March change of mind (Plaza II), Judge Pollak delved deep into the history of fingerprints, schooling himself on not only the minutiae of the science, but on the internal politics of the science (going so far as to criticize Winston Churchill for refusing to recognize Henry Faulds's foundational work in the field of friction-ridge analysis). In addition to his library research, the judge also called expert witnesses representing both sides of the fingerprint argument, questioning them himself from the bench for three days. At the conclusion of his fact finding, the judge found that while fingerprint specialists are not "scientists," they are "like accountants, vocational experts, accident-reconstruction experts, . . . [and] experts in tire failure analysis" possessed of "technical or other specialized knowledge" as required by Rule 702 (*United States v. Plaza* 2002, pp. 563–564).[15] After resolving the "science" issue, Judge Pollak next tackled the problem of a known error rate. Government experts had responded to his questions about error rates by offering proficiency test scores as a proxy. FBI fingerprint examiners – the focus of the motion to exclude – "scored spectacularly well on the in-house annual proficiency tests," and by interpolation, their actual error rate could be inferred to be low. This may not have been the strongest argument in favor of fingerprint analysis, but by contrast, the defense offered no counter evidence, and Judge Pollak was forced to conclude that "there is no evidence that the error rate of certified FBI fingerprint examiners is unacceptably high" (*United States v. Plaza* 2002, p. 566). Lastly, the judge addressed the matter of "testing." It was the one *Daubert* factor that remained in his opinion "both pertinent and unsatisfied," and he found no acceptable workaround. Nevertheless, the *Daubert* factors were never intended to be an exhaustive or mandatory list, and Judge Pollak found that, the testing issue notwithstanding, he was prepared to allow the opinion into evidence. He was not, upon reconsideration, "persuaded that courts should defer admission of testimony with respect to fingerprinting . . . until academic investigators financed by the National Institute of Justice have made substantial headway on a 'verification and validation' research agenda" (*United States v. Plaza* 2002, p. 572).

The opinion from *Plaza* exemplifies the difficulty of the "gatekeeper" role imposed upon trial judges. In the absence of reported statistical uncertainty (or certainty), the judge turned to proficiency exams to extrapolate a known error rate. Proficiency is the ability and/or capacity to do something to a prescribed level of mastery, which does not speak to the scientific validity and reliability of a method. In all fairness, there should be limited criticism for this decision considering that method validity falls under the practice of good science; meaning that criticism resides in the disciplines that promote poorly developed or non-validated methods.

## 2.8 Fear, reality, and forensic anthropology

While the courts grappled with the aftermath of the *Daubert* opinion, Forensic Anthropology was emerging from a transitional period punctuated by the broadening of its scope and a realization that the discipline was no longer considered simply the application of physical anthropological analyses to the medico-legal setting. The belief that analytical methods applied to the forensic context must meet specific demands owing to the potential evidentiary nature of the results brought about a renaissance in method validation. Furthermore, in the wake of the *Daubert* rulings, many forensic disciplines had begun to critically evaluate methods currently used for their examinations in fear of being confronted with an admissibility hearing. According to Lesciotto (2015), from 2004 to 2013 approximately 40 articles referencing *Daubert* in conjunction with method evaluation appear in the Anthropology section of the *Journal of Forensic Sciences*. Interest in method validation was likely fueled by the *Plaza* opinion considering the uptick in the early 2000s, which kicked into overdrive after the NAS report in 2009.

When strictly looking at the number of cases from 1975 to 2013 where federal and state courts examined the admissibility of Forensic Anthropology testimony, there is a distinct increase over time (Lesciotto 2015). A total of 277 cases were identified that mentioned Forensic Anthropology evidence and, of that number, only 30 cases evaluated the admissibility of Forensic Anthropology testimony. A large percentage of the identified cases involved analyses that are not typically within the anthropology analytical scope (i.e. footprint/shoeprint and photographic comparison analyses) and, therefore, the use of these methods was likely already controversial within the field. The overall low number of cases identified may have resulted from admissibility questions being raised and dismissed prior to a formal hearing or it simply reflects the infrequency of anthropologists testifying considering that the forensic pathologist often incorporates anthropological results into the report of autopsy findings. Regardless, in the decade following the *Daubert* rulings, the fear of admissibility hearings did not appear to be substantial enough to produce rapid change within Forensic Anthropology. Furthermore, the aforementioned infrequency of anthropologists providing expert testimony likely reduced the overall impact that the *Daubert* decision had on the field in the late 1990s and early 2000s.

## 2.9   The gauntlet is thrown: the NAS gets involved

It is entirely possible that "the power of the Supreme Court's *Daubert* decision was not so much in its formal doctrinal test, but rather in its ability to create greater awareness of the problems of junk science," and that "the practical merits and drawbacks of adopting a *Frye* versus a *Daubert* standard are largely superfluous" (Cheng and Yoon 2005, p. 503). That may in fact be the case, but the matter was soon to be further complicated by events happening in Hollywood.

## 2.10   The CSI effect

Certainly, police procedurals have been a mainstay of television from its earliest days, but it was perhaps the popularity of *Quincy, M.E.,* that made forensic science the successful plot device that it is today. Actor Jack Klugman's portrayal of the Los Angeles Medical Examiner captivated NBC audiences from 1976 to 1983 and for many viewers the show provided the first real glimpse into the existence of the medico-legal profession. What *Quincy, M.E.,* did not do, however, was fundamentally reshape the legal profession. That would have to wait until 2000 and the airing of a program with the almost documentary-like title: *CSI: Crime Scene Investigation*.

One of the earliest, if not the first, references to the term "CSI Effect" appeared in an October 2002 article in *Time* magazine (Kluger 2002). By 2005 the term was in widespread use, peaking a year or two later (Cole and Dioso-Villa 2007). Defined broadly, the CSI Effect is the creation of "unrealistic expectations among jurors" that "forensic, rather than circumstantial evidence, constantly solves crimes" (Cole and Dioso-Villa 2007, p. 441). The CSI Effect can operate in one of two ways (Cole and Dioso-Villa 2007).[16] Awareness of forensic techniques gleaned from television shows can raise the prosecutorial bar, i.e. jurors can come to expect that more can be done with crime-scene evidence – and should be done. But, conversely, and perhaps more perniciously, jurors can come to place too great a reliance on the power of forensic science, i.e. if the science says it is so, then it must be so. Therein lies the danger posed by a flawed forensic system. The *effect* of the "effect" was a hotly debated topic in the legal community for several years, with some scholars arguing that the popularity of forensic-science television shows has created an environment where a large segment of the population blindly assumes that "forensic scientists are actually practicing and engaging in legitimate science," while at the other end of the spectrum, attorneys, judges, and academics exhibit "an unprecedented level of skepticism and angst" about the state of the profession (Cooley 2011, p. 471). Certainly, there is some evidence that "viewers with a regular diet of forensic-science television" come to "regularly expect better science than what they often are presented with in courts," (Schweitzer and Saks 2007) though there is less evidence that this expectation affects trial outcome (Feeler 2014).

But while trial outcomes may or may not be overtly affected by the public's inundation with technology, there can be little doubt that jurors are nonetheless influenced by advances that are "part of a larger transformation occurring in popular and technological culture" (Shelton et al. 2006, p. 333). While many forensic practitioners jeer at pop-culture portrayal of forensic science, Shelton et al. (2006) suggest that it is incumbent upon the criminal justice system to adapt to these expectations of scientific evidence, rather than criticize or question them.

## 2.11  The congressional response

At the same time that public awareness was being piqued by the growth of CSI-related television programs, the nightly news was painting a picture of a forensic profession rotting from within. In early 2003, parts of the Houston Crime Lab collapsed in scandal; the Washington State Police Crime Lab suffered a similar public airing of its soiled laundry; and then, on March 11, 2004, terrorists detonated a series of bombs on several commuter trains in Madrid. Spanish police soon focused their attention on a van found near the train station that contained detonators and explosives, and a digital copy of a fingerprint found on one of the detonators was sent to the FBI for analysis. The FBI's vaunted fingerprint lab reported a match between the latent print and prints on file for an American lawyer living in Portland, Oregon, Brandon Mayfield. Mayfield was arrested but later released when the results of the fingerprint analysis where shown to be in error. The resulting investigation by the Department of Justice into what went wrong with the case found multiple points of failure in the FBI system (Department of Justice 2006).

Like stars aligning, these cracks in the forensic-science profession were developing at exactly the same time that television was raising popular awareness (and expectation) of forensic science and the lingering smell of junk science was still fresh in the public's nostrils. And the Supreme Court's response to the developing problem was anemic at best, pushing the matter back onto the robed shoulders of trial judges with the admonition to be better "gatekeepers." It was something akin to instructing a company headed for bankruptcy that its accountants should be better "bookkeepers."

Into this vacuum stepped Congress, and the result was the 2009 NAS report. Congress might not be able to affect change once the science was introduced in the courtroom, but it could have an effect on the quality of science before it ever got to the courthouse steps. How much impact the concept of the CSI Effect had on shaping the NAS report is not certain. What is clear is that in a post-*Daubert* world, forensic science could not expect the traditional hall pass that had always been granted. The NAS report took specific note of this changed environment. "The true effects of the popularization of forensic science disciplines will not be fully understood for some time, but it is apparent that it has increased pressure and attention on the forensic science community in the use and interpretation of evidence in the courtroom" (National Research Council 2009, p. 49).

## 2.12   The forensic sciences respond

The scientific community's reaction to the NAS report was swift compared with its rather sluggish response to the challenges posed by *Daubert*. In September of 2009 (American Academy of Forensic Sciences 2009), only seven months after the publication of the NAS report, the American Academy of Forensic Sciences (AAFS) released a position statement detailing its response. In this report the AAFS embraced the recommendations and provided the following principles the Academy endorses and promotes (www.aafs.org):

1. All forensic science disciplines must have a strong scientific foundation.
2. All forensic science laboratories should be accredited.
3. All forensic scientists should be certified.

4. Forensic science terminology should be standardized.
5. Forensic scientists should be assiduously held to Codes of Ethics.
6. Existing forensic science professional entities should participate in governmental oversight of the field.
7. Attorneys and judges who work with forensic scientists and forensic science evidence should have a strong awareness and knowledge of the scientific method and forensic science disciplines.

Note that six out of seven principles are speaking directly to the scientific community, providing a check list for getting their house in order. Two of the principles address quality assurance of practitioners and laboratories (see Chapter 5 for further discussion regarding QA/QC.) The final principle speaks to educating the legal community to assist the courts with the gatekeeper role, suggesting that testimony based on validated methods could still suffer if attorneys and judges are ill-informed.

Following the 2009 NAS report, federal funding programs became available and solicitations emphasized the importance of method development, validation, bias assessment, etc., specifically citing recommendations from the report. With the coffers open, research projects and published literature began frequently discussing *Daubert* and the NAS report. Currently, the anthropology literature has become inundated with researchers suggesting their method meets the *Daubert* criteria, seemingly providing more weight to its acceptance. This is a misunderstanding of how the gatekeeper role works and assumes that if research is conceived in the spirit of *Daubert*, that it would automatically pass any admissibility challenge. This creates a false sense of security, considering that the determination may differ case by case. A *Daubert* challenge by two different courts evaluating a similar scientific methodology may come to very different conclusions. Christensen et al. (2014) inform us that the NAS report reminds us to conduct good science so that, if challenged, it could pass the reliability aspect of the standard. Thus, the impetus for research is not to meet the *Daubert* standard, but to perform rigorous work because that is what we do as scientists. In a sense, the need for the judge to be the gatekeeper of "junk science" in the courtroom demonstrates a breakdown in the practice of science and indicates that some forensic practitioners have little or no understanding of the scientific method.

## 2.13   Picking up the gauntlet

In 2013, the Department of Justice (DOJ) established the National Commission on Forensic Science (NCFS), in partnership with the National Institute of Standards and Technology (NIST), to bolster the validity of the forensic sciences. In 2014, the Organization of Scientific Area Committees (OSAC) was developed and tasked with the development of best practice guidelines and standards for multiple forensic disciplines (Pierce et al. 2016). Prior to the release of the NAS report, Forensic Anthropology and other disciplines had already begun the process of determining best practices and developing consensus standards for the field. In 2008, a Scientific Working Group for Forensic Anthropology (SWGANTH) co-sponsored by the Department of Defense Joint POW/MIA Accounting Command and the FBI began the arduous task of developing and publishing best practices for the field. Thus, Forensic Anthropology was positioned well for the NCFS endeavor and the OSAC Anthropology subcommittee has leveraged the previous work.

Another pursuit within the field that is in line with the AAFS position statement is the accreditation of Forensic Anthropology laboratories and incorporation of the International Organization for Standardization (ISO) standards. Until recently, Anthropology was not a recognized field for accreditation programs (see Pierce et al. 2016 for information regarding the history of the accreditation program for Anthropology). As a result, there are many aspects of the practice of Forensic Anthropology that lacked demonstrative credibility to the community. According to Pierce et al. (2016):

> All forensic practitioners have the responsibility to ensure their opinions and testimonies are based on sound science, ethical practices, and transparent operations. The ISO standards have always fostered these objectives, and now avenues exist for forensic practitioners in the medico-legal setting to become accredited to those standards (p. 348).

As more Anthropology laboratories move toward accreditation and practitioners seek certification from the American Board of Forensic Anthropology (or other certification body), the discipline will have stronger scientific and procedural footings within the courts.

## 2.14  Conclusions

In reviewing the impetus for the NAS report and the initial impact and response in the forensic sciences, specifically in Forensic Anthropology, we started with the question: "How did we get here?" but we end with the question: "Now that we are here, where do we go next?"

The first question is simple, we got here because the legal system trusted scientists to police ourselves, and we broke that trust. *Frye's* General Acceptance test ensured that only science that had been vetted by time and practice was allowed into the courtroom. That type of self-regulation worked for almost 70 years, but in the years following World War Two, when science was advancing at an ever-increasing pace, the system began to break down, making it vulnerable to the greed that came to characterize the toxic-tort era. Scientists, and those posing as scientists, were not immune to that greed, and in response to the ensuing "junk science" the Supreme Court installed the trial judge in the role of the gatekeeper – the housemother in the frat house. And the gatekeeper brought a checklist of criteria that the NAS nailed to the front door.

And that is where we are, and how we got here.

The second question is a bit more nuanced. The NAS report makes scant reference to Forensic Anthropology (only six times in 328 pages, including the index entry). That may be because Forensic Anthropology, at least in the big forensic picture, plays a small role, but it may also be because we are already doing a good job at the science part of the problem. Forensic Anthropology is strongly rooted in its science, and in fact, the practical application of anthropology to legal matters is a relatively recent development. Because of these firm roots, Forensic Anthropology hasn't strayed too far from home and is still taught largely as a science first, and a practical application second. By contrast, some of the other forensic "sciences" have been application oriented for so long, that their scientific roots are barely recognizable; the underlying science lost and forgotten to its practitioners today. For example, there is no doubt that fingerprinting – the archetype of forensic science – had its beginning strongly rooted in science,[17] but it quickly became a formulaic application in forensics that took the foundational science for granted. Over time, that foundation was lost, at least until *Llera Plaza*. For these sub-disciplines, the NAS report was a clear call to rediscover their roots.

But Forensic Anthropology never forgot its roots. Forensic Anthropology has the opposite problem. Its science is largely sound, but as a profession it is less comfortable with the language and procedure of the courtroom. Anthropologists who are fluent in the mechanics of R-values and confidence intervals chaff at the notion that they may have to follow a lab SOP, or work in the blind, or take their notes in a certain color of ink. The same people who willingly sat for five-day qualifying examinations and three-hour dissertation defenses, draw the line at annual proficiency testing, and board certification, and lab accreditation. This is the challenge facing us as a profession: we must learn to speak the language of forensics.

The good news is that we are starting to make progress. Groups such as the SWGANTH, and now the OSAC subcommittee for Anthropology, are striving to establish best practices and procedural standards. Forensic Anthropology laboratories are beginning to seek accreditation and pressure is mounting for those that are failing to react, and method development in the literature incorporates more in-depth statistical analyses and trends for error analysis are increasing. The discussions are shifting from *"why do we need accreditation?"* to *"what should the accreditation encompass?"* That is a major step in the right direction.

There is no doubt that Forensic Science, writ large, was lackadaisical in policing itself, allowing the generalization of the term "science" and the illusion that invoking the term "forensic science" somehow imbued the various fields with unquestionable validity. Since the *Daubert* rulings and the NAS report, Forensic Anthropology has slowly begun to embrace the concepts of quality assurance and lab accreditation. It is through quality assurance and the practice of good science that our field will provide a durable structure to answer the call from the courts for valid and reliable forensic science. While accreditation and certification will not clarify the gatekeeper role for trial judges, it will help to illuminate that *twilight zone* where the evidential force of the scientific principle must be recognized.

## Notes

1. Professor Starrs accessed the available original trial records form the case and conducted an interview with Frye's widow. Based on his analysis of the case, Starrs concluded that James Frye likely was guilty of Dr. Brown's murder, despite what his blood pressure might otherwise have indicated.
2. An Act to Establish Rules of Evidence for Certain Courts and Proceedings, Pub L. No. 93-595, 88 Stat 1926. Rule 1101 makes the FRE applicable to "United States district courts; United States bankruptcy and magistrate judges; United States courts of appeals; the United States Court of Federal Claims; and the district courts of Guam, the Virgin Islands, and the Northern Mariana Islands."
3. The first major civil suit in which the term "Toxic Tort" appears is In re Agent Orange Products Liability Litigation, 506 F. Supp. 737 (E.D.N.Y. 1979), *rev'd*, 635 F.2d 987 (2d Cir. 1980), *cert denied*, 454 U.S. 1128 (1981).
4. Many more cases were settled out of court. One of the more famous examples being the $333 million settlement by Pacific Gas and Electric Company to the inhabitants of Hinkley, CA, made popular by the movie *Erin Brockovich*.
5. By 1993 the four major implant manufacturers – Dow Corning, Bristol-Myers Squibb, Baxter Healthcare, and 3M – had set aside $4.75 billion for the purposing of paying out potential claims (Fisher, 2015).
6. Johns-Manville Corporation had been one of the largest manufacturers of asbestos products. Mesothelioma lawsuits forced the company into Chapter 11 in 1982. Similarly, A.H. Robbins marked the intrauterine device (IUD) known as the Dalkon Shield. Lawsuits by users of the device resulted in A.H. Robbins filing for Chapter 11 in 1985.
7. Dow Corning and Merrell Dow Pharmaceuticals involve corporate spin-offs from the parent organization, Dow Chemical, which holds the dubious honor of having its name associated with both the silicone breast-implant cases and the Bendectin cases.
8. The flames also were fanned by a 1990 airing of a *Face to Face with Connie Chung* episode on NBC that highlighted unsubstantiated claims of illnesses caused by silicone exposure, and which Jack Fisher has termed "a new low for one-sided fearmongering journalism" (Fisher 2015).
9. The pronunciation of "Daubert" has occasionally been a point of discussion. The lead attorney for the Daubert family clarified the confusion in a 1994 article in which he

stated that the family pronounces the name as if it were "Dow-burt," rather than "Dough-bear." The confusion didn't start with the Supreme Court, but was exacerbated during oral argument when the first Justice to ask a question pronounced it "Dough-bear" and the other Justices followed suit (Gottesman 1994).

10. Numerous epidemiological studies conducted at the time found no such association between Bendectin use and birth defects; nonetheless, by the early 1980s Dow's cost of defending lawsuits had made the continued marketing of Bendectin unprofitable (Brody 1993).

11. The case originally was brought in a state court in California but was removed to the United States Court for the Southern District of California at the request of Dow Pharmaceuticals on the grounds that the Dow Corporation was a "resident" of Delaware and the plaintiffs were residents of California.

12. Not all of the Justices believed these general observations would prove workable in specific cases. Chief Justice Rehnquist, while concurring with the opinion that the FRE superseded *Frye*, dissented with the majority's adoption of the general principles. While there is a requirement for "some gatekeeping responsibility" on the part of judges, Rehnquist feared that the Court's general observations ran the risk of imposing on judges "either the obligation or the authority to become amateur scientists in order to perform that role" (Daubert 1993).

13. A third case often cited as part of the "*Daubert* trilogy" is *Kumho Tire Co. v. Carmichael*, 526 U.S. 137 (1999). Kumho Tire extended Daubert's reach to include technical and engineering expertise in addition to scientific.

14. *Llera Plaza* was not the first case to challenge fingerprinting in the post-*Daubert* era but is notable for the level of insight provided by the judge in how the opinion was reached. One of the first cases to review fingerprints under the requirements of the FRE, *United States v. Harvard* (2000), not only found that fingerprinting met the *Daubert* criteria, but went on to state that "latent print identification is the very archetype of reliable expert testimony under those standards." (see generally Cole 2004).

15. The reference to "tire failure analysis" invokes the central issue of *Kumho Tire Co. v. Carmichael,* which expanded *Daubert* to apply to technical specialties.

16. Cole and Dioso-Villa argue that there are actually six different CSI Effects, operating on jurors, prosecutors, criminals, and prospective students of forensic science.

17. Ironically, most of the early, and for that matter on-going, work on friction-ridge science and dermatoglyphics has been done by anthropologists. Sir Francis Galton generally is regarded as the father of academic fingerprint study. His seminal work, "Finger Prints," was first published in 1892, but it was developed from a lecture given four years earlier at the Royal Institution. (Galton 1892; see also Galton 1888).

# References

American Academy of Forensic Sciences. The American Academy of Forensic Sciences Approves Position Statement in Response to the National Academy of Sciences' "Forensic Needs" Report: Academy News (2009). https://news.aafs.org/policy-statements/the-american-academy-of-forensic-sciences-approves-position-statement-in-response-to-the-national-academy-of-sciences-forensic-needs-report (accessed September 25, 2018).

Becker, E.R. and Orenstein, A. (1992). The Federal Rules of Evidence after sixteen years — the effect of "plain meaning" jurisprudence, the need for an advisory committee on the rules of evidence, and suggestions for selective revision of the rules. *George Washington Law Review* 60: 857–914.

Billauer, B.P. (2016). Daubert debunked: a history of legal retrogression and the need to reassess "scientific admissibility". *Suffolk Journal of Trial and Appellate Advocacy* 21: 1–57.

Brody, J.E. (1993). Shadow of a doubt wipes out Bendectin. *New York Times*. http://www.nytimes.com/1983/06/19/weekinreview/shadow-of-doubt-wipes-out-bendectin.html (accessed June 28, 2017).

Cheng, E.K. and Yoon, A.H. (2005). Does Fyre or Daubert matter? A study of scientific admissibility standards. *Virginia Law Review* 91: 471–513.

Christensen, A., Crowder, C., Ousley, S., and Houck, M.M. (2014). Errors and its meaning in forensic science. *Journal of Forensic Science* 59 (1): 123–126.

Cole, S.A. (2004). Grandfathering evidence: fingerprint admissibility rulings from Jennings to Llera Plaza and back again. *American Criminal Law Review* 41: 1189–1276.

Cole, S.A. and Dioso-Villa, R. (2007). CSI and its effects: media, juries, and the burden of proof. *New England Law Review* 41: 435–469.

Confesses to Murder *Confesses to murder of Colored physician*. *Evening Star* (August 231921), p. 5. http://chroniclingamerica.loc.gov/lccn/sn83045462/1921-08-23/ed-1/seq-5 (accessed June 28, 2017).

Cooley, C.M. (2011). The CSI effect: the true effect of crime scene television on the justice system. *New England Law Review* 41: 471–501.

*Daubert v. Merrell Dow Pharmaceuticals*, 727 F. Supp 570 (S.D. Cal. 1989).

*Daubert v. Merrell Dow Pharmaceuticals*, 951 F.2d 1128 (9th Cir. 1991).

*Daubert v. Merrell Dow Pharmaceuticals, Inc.*, 509 U.S. 579 (1993)

Department of Justice, Office of the Inspector General, (2006). Special Report: A Review of the FBI's Handling of the Brandon Mayfield Case. [Unclassified and Redacted Version]. https://oig.justice.gov/special/s0601/PDF_list.htm (accessed November 12, 2017).

Dixon, L. and Gill, B. (2001). *Changes in the Standards for Admitting Expert Evidence in Federal Civil Cases Since the Daubert Decision*. Santa Monica: RAND Institute for Civil Justice.

Duchesnay Inc. Bendectin history. 2017 http://www.bendectin.com/en (accessed June 28, 2017).

Feeler, W. (2014). Can fiction impede conviction? Addressing claims of a "CSI effect" in the criminal courtroom. *Mississippi Law Journal* 83: 1–57.

Fisher, J.C. (2015). *Silicone on Trial*. Sager Group.

Frontline, WGBH Educational Foundation. (n.d.)Chronology of silicone breast implants. http://www.pbs.org/wgbh/pages/frontline/implants/cron.html (accessed October 26, 2017).

*Frye v. United States*, 293 F. 1013 (D.C. Cir. 1923).

Galton, F. (1888). Personal identification and description. *Nature* 38: 173, 201–177, 202.

Galton, F. (1892). Finger prints. http://galton.org/books/finger-prints/galton-1892-fingerprints-1up-lowres.pdf (accessed May 15, 2017).

*General Electric v. Joiner*. (1997). 522 U.S. 136.

Giannelli, P.C. (1994). Daubert: interpreting the Federal Rules of evidence. *Cardozo Law Review* 15: 1999–2026.

Godden, D.M. and Walton, D. (2006). Argument from expert opinion as legal evidence: critical questions and admissibility criteria of expert testimony in the American legal system. *Ratio Juris* 19: 261–286.

Gottesman, M.H. (1994). Admissibility of expert testimony after Daubert: the "prestige" factor. *Emory Law Journal* 43: 867.

Huber, P.W. (1993). *Galileo's Revenge: Junk Science in the Courtroom*. New York: Basic Books.

In re Air Crash Disaster at New Orleans, 795 F.2d 1230 (5th Cir. 1986).

Institute of Medicine (US) Committee on the Safety of Silicone Breast Implants (1999). Executive Summary. https://www.ncbi.nlm.nih.gov/books/NBK44778 (accessed November 1, 2017).

Kluger, J., (2002). How science solves crimes. *Time* (October 21), p. 36.

*Kumho Tire Co. v. Carmichael*, 526 U.S. 137 (1999).

Lepore, J. (2015a). On evidence: proving Frye as a matter of law, science, and history. *Yale Law Journal* 124: 1092–1158.

Lepore, J. (2015b). *The Secret History of Wonder Woman*. New York: Vintage.

Lesciotto, K.M. (2015). The impact of Daubert on the admissibility of forensic anthropology expert testimony. *Journal of Forensic Sciences* 60: 549–555.

National Research Council (2009). *Strengthening Forensic Science in the United States: A Path Forward*. Washington, DC: National Academies Press.

*People v. Jennings*, 96 N.E. 1077 (IL 1911).

Pierce, M.L., Wiersema, J.M., and Crowder, C.M. (2016). Progress in the accreditation of anthropology laboratories. *Academic Forensic Pathology* 6 (3): 344–348.

Schweitzer, N.J. and Saks, M.J. (2007). The CSI effect: popular fiction about forensic science affects the public's expectations about real forensic science. *Jurimetrics* 47: 357–364.

Shelton, D.E., Kim, Y.S., and Barak, G. (2006). A study of juror expectations and demands concerning scientific evidence: does the 'CSI Effect' exist? *Vanderbilt Journal of Entertainment & Technology Law* 9: 330–368.

Slain in Home. Slain in his home by unknown man. *Sunday [Evening] Star* [Washington DC] (November 28 1920), p. 1. http://chroniclingamerica.loc.gov/lccn/sn83045462/1920-11-28/ed-1/seq-1 (accessed June 28, 2017).

Starrs, J.E. (1982). "A still-life watercolor": Frye v. United States. *Journal of Forensic Sciences* 27: 684–694.

Studebaker, C.L. and Goodman-Delahunty, J. (eds.) (2002). Special theme: expert testimony in the courts: the influence of the Daubert, Joiner, and Kumho decisions, part 1: hindsight bias, Daubert, and the silicone breast implant litigation: making the case for court-appointed experts in complex medical and scientific litigation. *Psychology, Public Policy, and Law* 8: 154–178.

United States (1975). The federal rules of evidence [Rule 702]. Albany, NY: Matthew Bender.

*United States v. Harvard*, 117 F. Supp, 848, 855 (S.D. Ind. 2000).

*United States v. Plaza*, 188 F. Supp. 2d 549 (E.D. Pa. 2002).

*V. Mueller & Co. v. Corley*, 570 S.W.2d 140 (Tex. App. 1978).

# CHAPTER 3

# From the laboratory to the witness stand: research trends and method validation in forensic anthropology

Jonathan D. Bethard[1] and Elizabeth A. DiGangi[2]

[1] University of South Florida, Tampa, FL, USA
[2] Binghamton University, Binghamton, NY, USA

> The researcher considers her or himself to be a forensic scientist first, with knowledge and expertise of relevance to a particular case, in other words an EXPERT witness. In actuality he or she is an instrument of the retaining attorney and the courts, i.e. an expert WITNESS.
>
> *Bird 2001, p. 979*

## 3.1   Introduction

Forensic Anthropologists are routinely asked to contribute to medico-legal investigations through their analyses of human skeletal and dental tissues. Beyond providing information about a decedent's biological profile, Forensic Anthropologists are often charged with providing their expertise on matters relating to skeletal trauma analysis and the postmortem interval. The process of generating a report for a coroner, medical examiner, or other interested stakeholder requires the Forensic Anthropologist to draw from a large body of published literature while applying this diverse information to the skeletonized human remains on the laboratory table. However, the incorporation of relevant research into case reports varies among practitioners; and no nationally adopted guidelines provide specific instructions on how to approach this process in medico-legal contexts in the United States.

In some instances, the Forensic Anthropology report becomes of evidentiary value in a court proceeding, requiring the anthropologist to function as an expert witness. In this situation, the Forensic Anthropology witness is charged with relaying their findings to a group of laypeople with little or no expertise in the subject under discussion. As Bird (2001) notes, the presentation of findings in the courtroom varies substantially from how findings are relayed in the research arena. Academic conference presentations, peer-reviewed journal articles, and invited book chapters are common platforms for a Forensic Anthropologist to present their research to an interested audience of other anthropologists or interested specialists; however, the environment of the courtroom requires them to convey information and present an authoritative opinion about the scientific certainty of the evidence related to a particular case in a way that is decidedly different from a conference presentation or peer-reviewed publication (Bird 2001). In addition, the testimony of the Forensic Anthropologist may only focus on one aspect of a case and the other analyses completed (e.g. age, ancestry, or stature estimates) may not be of interest in the courtroom. For example, a *Daubert*-compliant forensic anthropological sex assessment may not be discussed at trial because a positive identification of the victim may have been already established by other means or an explanation about the etiology of a cutmark may be of more significant evidentiary value (see Chapter 2 for more on *Daubert*). In this example therefore, the bulk of the forensic anthropological literature as well as other areas of research may be of little importance to the courtroom proceeding.

How Forensic Anthropologists translate research drawn from biological anthropology, archaeology, biomechanics, human anatomy and other scholarly disciplines into courtroom testimony is admittedly challenging. This chapter discusses the link between research and the courtroom in US-based forensic anthropological contexts. In addition, this chapter highlights the emerging incongruity between research focused on the biological profile and the areas which often require forensic anthropological testimony: namely, skeletal trauma analysis and estimation of the postmortem interval.

The inconsistencies between forensic anthropological research and courtroom testimony trends have received little attention by the forensic anthropological community in the United States; however, some discussion about the variable use of language has been initiated (Bunch 2014). As noted by Bunch (2014), the different meaning ascribed to the term *perimortem* by forensic pathologists is somewhat variable from how Forensic Anthropologists utilize the term. Moreover, Bunch (2014) notes Forensic Anthropologists define *perimortem* in slightly different ways despite a sweeping movement for standardization across the discipline. Though the concept of *perimortem* has posed challenges for Forensic Anthropologists, discussions about terminology have spurred research incorporating bone biomechanics with skeletal trauma analysis (Symes et al. 2014, Kroman and Symes 2013).

The emphasis of research related to the biological profile has recently been described in the literature by Lesciotto (2015), who also noted the discrepancy between research trends and courtroom testimony. This publication represents the first, and perhaps only, contribution discussing the admissibility of Forensic Anthropology testimony in the United States by data mining published court decisions. Drawing on her legal training, Lesciotto (2015) utilized the search engines *LexisNexis Academic* and *Daubert Tracker* to access decisions from all federal and state courts which included the phrases "Forensic Anthropology" or "Forensic Anthropologist."

Lesciotto (2015) assembled a sample of 333 court cases spanning the temporal period 1975–2013 and documented that forensic anthropological evidence consisted of 40% skeletal trauma analysis, 19% biological profile or victim identification, and 11% postmortem interval estimation. The remaining types of forensic anthropological evidence included diverse topics such as forensic recovery, footprint analysis, and photographic comparisons (Lesciotto 2015). These types of evidence were also tracked by temporal period and demonstrate that skeletal trauma represents over 50% of the testimony for the most recent temporal period in the study (i.e. 2010–2013) and are even more prominent in the period 2010–2017 (Lesciotto 2015; K. Lesciotto, personal communication, 2017). Lesciotto (2015) notes that admissibility challenges to forensic anthropological evidence have been relatively infrequent in the post-*Daubert* era, and argues that the field has stayed ahead of legal requirements related to admissibility challenges.

While Lesciotto (2015) has demonstrated that skeletal trauma is the most common type of evidence presented in the courtroom as forensic anthropological testimony, methodological rigor is compulsory. Numerous contributions have explicitly tackled topics such as defining "error" and have reiterated the importance of validation studies in relation to the biological profile and/or techniques utilized to establish a positive identification (Christensen et al. 2014; Christensen and Crowder 2009; Christensen 2004; Budowle et al. 2009; Steadman et al. 2006).

## 3.2  Research in forensic anthropology – a bibliometric survey

Drawing on Lesciotto (2015) who documents a publication surge toward more objective and quantifiable techniques in response to *Daubert*, the authors conducted a bibliometric survey to understand general trends related to forensic anthropological research published in the *Journal of Forensic Sciences* (*JFS*) from January 2000 to July 2018. *JFS* contributions in the "Physical Anthropology" or

**Table 3.1** Topical breakdown of Anthropology contributions published in the *Journal of Forensic Sciences* from January 2000 to July 2018.

|  | Frequency | Percent |
| --- | --- | --- |
| Biological profile | 300 | 39.5 |
| Taphonomic studies/Postmortem interval estimation | 104 | 13.7 |
| Skeletal trauma analysis | 73 | 9.6 |
| Facial approximation | 61 | 8 |
| Positive identification | 54 | 7.1 |
| Histology/Bone anatomy/Bone identification | 21 | 2.8 |
| Human rights/Humanitarian issues | 21 | 2.8 |
| Field methods/Forensic archaeology | 19 | 2.5 |
| Isotopes/Elemental composition | 17 | 2.2 |
| DNA analyses | 16 | 2.1 |
| History | 16 | 2.1 |
| Osteometrics/Laboratory procedures | 15 | 2 |
| Skeletal pathology | 11 | 1.4 |
| Commingling | 10 | 1.3 |
| Processing/Maceration | 7 | 0.9 |
| Legal issues | 7 | 0.9 |
| Ethics/Theory | 6 | 0.8 |
| Secular change | 2 | 0.3 |
| **Total** | 760 | 100 |

"Anthropology" categories were included along with a small number of relevant papers published under other sections of the American Academy of Forensic Sciences (AAFS) (e.g. Megyesi et al. 2005 was published by the Pathology/Biology section). Contributions included Papers, Technical Notes, and Case Reports and were categorized by topic (e.g. biological profile, skeletal trauma analysis, taphonomy, facial approximation, etc., see Table 3.1). Additionally, papers falling into the biological profile category were further divided into topical areas of research (e.g. sex estimation or age estimation, see Table 3.2). The aim of this bibliometric survey is to provide the readership of this volume with data summarizing forensic anthropological research trends and how knowledge of these trends can inform or could contribute to the improvement of forensic anthropological testimony in the courtroom.

Seven hundred and sixty contributions were published during the queried period. Since 2000, contributions related to Forensic Anthropology in *JFS* have steadily increased in number (see Figure 3.1).

**Table 3.2** Breakdown of topics focused on the biological profile published in the *Journal of Forensic Sciences* from January 2000 to July 2018.

|  | Frequency | Percent |
|---|---|---|
| Age | 119 | 39.7 |
| Sex | 112 | 37.3 |
| Ancestry | 38 | 12.7 |
| Stature | 22 | 7.3 |
| Parturition | 3 | 1 |
| Body mass | 4 | 1.3 |
| Handedness | 2 | 0.7 |
| **Total** | 300 | 100 |

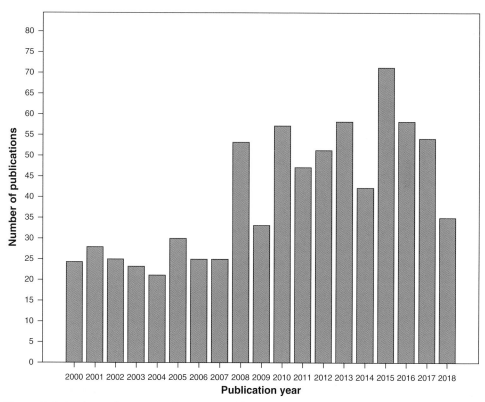

**Figure 3.1** Anthropology contributions published in the *Journal of Forensic Sciences* since 2000. Note that 2018 data is through the July issue.

The year 2004 is the year with the fewest number of papers published ($n = 21$) and 2015 has the most ($n = 71$). The year 2018 will likely top 50 contributions.

Turning to content, publications related to the biological profile represent 39.5% of contributions ($n = 300$), 13.7% ($n = 104$) are related to taphonomic studies or estimation of the postmortem interval, and 9.6% ($n = 73$) focus on skeletal trauma analysis (Table 3.1).

These three topical foci represent nearly 63% of Forensic Anthropology contributions published during the first two decades of the twenty-first century.

Of the 300 papers focused on the biological profile, 77.3% ($n = 231$) discuss either age estimation ($n = 119$) or sex estimation ($n = 112$) (Table 3.2).

Ancestry and stature are represented by relatively few contributions ($n = 60$) and a small number of publications discuss parturition, body mass estimation, or handedness.

What does this content analysis tell us about the status of forensic anthropological research published in *JFS*? We argue that this analysis demonstrates that research on at least two parameters of the biological profile is robust. Indeed, contributions related to the study of age estimation cover the entirety of the human lifespan ranging from the youngest fetal individuals (e.g. Adalian et al. 2001), older children and non-adults (e.g. Santana et al. 2017), and elderly individuals (e.g. Cappella et al. 2017). Contributions related to sex estimation thoroughly cover methodological approaches derived from the pelvis, post-cranial skeleton, and cranial morphology (Fowler and Hughes 2018; Klales 2016; Lewis and Garvin 2016; Tallman and Go 2018); however, few if any publications in *JFS* or elsewhere have yet to tackle the issue of how a Forensic Anthropologist might provide information regarding the biological profile of an intersexed or transgendered decedent (Buchanan 2014; Jones 2014; Geller 2009). Given that there are over 12 000 individuals listed in the "Unidentified Persons" section of the National Missing and Unidentified Persons System (www.namus.gov), it is conceivable that discontinuities between biological parameters of the skeleton and self-reported identifiers are precluding positive identifications in some instances.

Areas of research related to the estimation of the other parameters of the biological profile (e.g. ancestry and stature) have been published much less frequently. Why this is remains somewhat unclear. However, in her doctoral dissertation, Parsons (2017) found that stature has little effect on the resolution of missing persons cases in large medical examiner's offices in the United States; therefore, we argue that this fact likely influences Forensic Anthropologists to pursue other areas of research besides stature estimation. In addition, Parsons (2017) found that FORDISC 3.1 misclassified ancestry estimates in 64% of cases of individuals who were positively identified as belonging to Hispanic populations in the United States. Recently Dudzik and Jantz (2016) reached a similar conclusion regarding the misclassification of Hispanic individuals with FORDISC 3.1. Though ancestry estimation has lagged behind in the number of publications compared with age and sex estimation, contributions such as those published by Dudzik and Jantz (2016) appear to have potentially energized research on this area of the biological profile.

Perhaps more problematic than the relative dearth of research on stature and ancestry estimation is the way in which research on the biological profile is far outpacing research in other areas of Forensic Anthropology. Given that Lesciotto (2015) has convincingly demonstrated that skeletal trauma and the postmortem interval are more likely to become important from an evidentiary standpoint, we argue that the bibliometric results presented in this chapter warrant some discussions about the demonstrated research trends in addition to the direction undergraduate and graduate training in Forensic Anthropology should take. Moreover, the National Institute of Justice (NIJ) Forensic Science Technology Working Group Operation Requirements for 2018 outlined multiple research needs within the forensic sciences. Several of these involve skeletal trauma analysis:

- "improved analysis and interpretation of sharp force trauma injuries on hard and soft tissues"
- "improved analysis and interpretation of blast/explosive trauma injuries" (https://www.nij.gov/topics/forensics/documents/2018-2-forensic-twg-table .pdf, p. 12, accessed 20 June 2018).

In addition, the Organization of Scientific Area Committees (OSAC) for Forensic Science Anthropology Subcommittee has also identified Research and Development Needs related to skeletal trauma analysis. Similar to the NIJ Technical Working Group, the OSAC Anthropology Subcommittee has published a Research and Development Needs document titled "Controlled Experimental Bone Trauma Studies" (https://www.nist.gov/document/ osacanthro1researchneedsbonetraumadocx, accessed 20 June 2018).

Despite the increased evidentiary importance of skeletal trauma analysis, as well as identified needs related to increased research on the topic, curriculum options and graduate courses in trauma analysis are variable and/or limited across graduate programs in the United States. In general, graduate students at different universities do not have the same curriculum offerings, faculty preferentially teach specific areas of the literature over others, and certain skillsets are difficult to acquire during graduate training (e.g. learning skeletal trauma analysis in the context of a medical examiner's office). New literature is also slow to enter casework standard operating procedures (SOPs) even after validation studies have been performed. For example, Garvin and Passalacqua (2012) highlighted the methods that are routinely utilized by Forensic Anthropologists for age estimation from the pubic symphysis. They observed that

27.9% of Forensic Anthropologists preferentially utilize Todd (1920) instead of newer methods derived from modern autopsy samples (e.g. Hartnett 2010). Finally, Bethard (2017) documents the diverse array of dissertation topics that board-certified Forensic Anthropologists pursued prior to achieving their Diplomate status from the American Board of Forensic Anthropology (ABFA). Bethard (2017) noted that a majority of board-certified Forensic Anthropologists conducted their doctoral work on research outside of Forensic Anthropology and that as of 2017, only one board-certified Forensic Anthropologist had conducted doctoral research related to skeletal trauma analysis.

## 3.3   Court decisions and research

As we have demonstrated throughout this chapter, the state of research in Forensic Anthropology overall is robust, with hundreds of contributions to the literature over the past 20 years. This is despite the field's relative youth and finite number of practitioners, especially compared with other areas of anthropology. What began as a strict application of knowledge from physical anthropology (e.g. Stewart 1979) has grown into a mature discipline complete with theoretical perspectives (Boyd and Boyd 2011, 2018). Initially, research in the field was focused on the biological profile, and as the field matured, scholars began exploring other topics such as trauma and taphonomy (Dirkmaat et al. 2008). However, the field was struck with a sense of urgency with the 1993 *Daubert v. Merrill Dow Pharmaceuticals, Inc*. Supreme Court decision.

Essentially, *Daubert* clarified that the Federal Rules of Evidence, laid out by Congress in 1975, superseded the earlier 1923 *Frye* standard of general acceptance with regards to evidence admissibility in federal court (see Chapters 1 and 2 for further discussion). In addition, the Supreme Court ruled that the judge is the gatekeeper of evidence and expert witness admission. There are four guidelines that judges must consider about the theory or technique: (1) whether it can be/has been tested; (2) whether it has been peer reviewed and published; (3) its known or potential error rate; and (4) its general acceptance. As a result of this decision Forensic Anthropologists grew concerned whether their expertise would be admissible in court, given that many of the methods used did not have error rates associated with them (e.g. Christensen 2004).

Consequently, a majority of papers since have focused on developing or revising methods so that they would comply with the *Daubert* standard. This approach is consistent with the current state of the law and the ability of Forensic Anthropologists to demonstrate reliable methodology. However, it remains that the majority of the expertise brought to bear by Forensic Anthropologists is not necessarily amenable to standardized methodology, and therefore does not fit squarely within the *Daubert* framework. For example, trauma analysis and taphonomy (with the exception of some postmortem interval methods) are primarily experience-based, subjective, and rely on pattern analysis. While ultimately grounded in scientific principles such as biomechanics, bone biology, and decomposition ecology, these analyses do not and cannot include error rates. A Forensic Anthropologist's ability to recognize an entrance gunshot wound versus an exit wound or to sequence the order of multiple cranial gunshot wounds is entirely based on their training and experience. Therefore, under a strict application of the *Daubert* standard, much forensic testimony would seemingly be subject to exclusion.

The Supreme Court addressed this gap in the admissibility of evidence based on training and technical expertise in its 1999 decision, *Kumho Tire v. Carmichael*. There, the Court clarified that such evidence may be admissible under *Daubert*, and that courts should evaluate the reliability of such evidence as part of their gatekeeping function. Thus, even absent standardized methods, forensic expertise may still be admissible. However, the process of assessing that expertise will be equally rigorous to the evaluation of empirical scientific evidence (Grivas and Komar 2008), and Forensic Anthropology must continue to maintain meticulous standard training/procedures/documentation and supporting data to ensure reliability. Grivas and Komar (2008) implore scholars to remember that *Kumho Tire* is the likely standard our work will be held to in federal court. Given that cases involving trauma testimony have steadily increased (Lesciotto 2015), Forensic Anthropologists should be cognizant that training in this area is particularly critical. While we should continue to produce vigorous research related to the biological profile, research in the realms of trauma analysis and taphonomy are just as important, if not more so.

## 3.4   Conclusion and a path forward

This chapter has provided Forensic Anthropologists with a useful summary of research trends over the last 20 years. Additionally, this chapter begins a conversation about the vexing courtroom reality facing Forensic Anthropologists today: testimony often focuses on areas of our specialized knowledge instead of our *Daubert*-centric research related to the biological profile.

From the work of Lesciotto (2015), as well as the bibliometric survey, a disconnect is presented between the current status of research and those areas most likely to become testimony. Fundamentally, a renewed emphasis on these areas of forensic anthropological scholarship considering the *Kumho* decision may simultaneously improve research and training. Though the authors appreciate the publication surge related to the *Daubert* narrative during the last two decades, the time has come to consider redirecting our research efforts toward the areas of evidentiary importance. This chapter underscores the importance that Forensic Anthropologists continue to conduct vigorous research related to the biological profile which provides error rates and is continually validated. However, the hope is that the information presented in this chapter will push the discipline to consider how some areas of Forensic Anthropology, namely skeletal trauma analysis and time since death estimation, would be best conceptualized as forms of pattern analysis which inherently rely on experimental studies and experience. As a result, both research and graduate training that have trauma and taphonomy as major foci are essential for a well-rounded education in Forensic Anthropology.

## Acknowledgments

We would like to thank Kate Lesciotto for her helpful comments and suggestions and for providing additional data regarding court cases utilizing forensic anthropological evidence. In addition, we thank the editors for inviting us to contribute this chapter to this important volume.

## References

Adalian, P., Piercecchi-Marti, M.D., Bourliere-Najean, B. et al. (2001). Postmortem assessment of fetal diaphyseal femoral length: validation of a radiographic methodology. *Journal of Forensic Sciences* 46 (2): 215–219.

Bethard, J.D. (2017). Historical trends in graduate research and training of Diplomates of the American Board of Forensic Anthropology. *Journal of Forensic Sciences* 62 (1): 5–11.

Bird, S.J. (2001). Scientific certainty: research versus forensic perspectives. *Journal of Forensic Sciences* 46 (4): 978–981.

Boyd, C. and Boyd, D.C. (2011). Theory and the scientific basis for forensic anthropology. *Journal of Forensic Sciences* 56 (6): 1407–1415.

Boyd, C.C. and Boyd, D.C. (2018). *Forensic Anthropology: Theoretical Framework and Scientific Basis*. John Wiley & Sons.

Buchanan, S. (2014). Bone modification in male to female transgender surgeries: considerations for the Forensic Anthropologist. MA thesis. Louisana State University.

Budowle, B., Bottrell, M.C., Bunch, S.G. et al. (2009). A perspective on errors, bias, and interpretation in the forensic sciences and direction for continuing advancement. *Journal of Forensic Sciences* 54 (4): 798–809.

Bunch, A.W. (2014). National Academy of Sciences "standardization": on what terms? *Journal of Forensic Sciences* 59 (4): 1041–1045.

Cappella, A., Cummaudo, M., Arrigoni, E. et al. (2017). The issue of age estimation in a modern skeletal population: are even the more modern current aging methods satisfactory for the elderly? *Journal of Forensic Sciences* 62 (1): 12–17.

Christensen, A.M. (2004). The impact of Daubert: implications for testimony and research in forensic anthropology (and the use of frontal sinuses in personal identification). *Journal of Forensic Sciences* 49 (3): 427–430.

Christensen, A.M. and Crowder, C.M. (2009). Evidentiary standards for forensic anthropology. *Journal of Forensic Sciences* 54 (6): 1211–1216.

Christensen, A.M., Crowder, C.M., Ousley, S.D., and Houck, M.M. (2014). Error and its
meaning in forensic science. *Journal of Forensic Sciences* 59 (1): 123–126.

Dirkmaat, D.C., Cabo, L.L., Ousley, S.D., and Symes, S.A. (2008). New perspectives in
forensic anthropology. *American Journal of Physical Anthropology* 137 (47): 33–52.

Dudzik, B. and Jantz, R.L. (2016). Misclassifications of Hispanics using Fordisc 3.1:
comparing cranial morphology in Asian and Hispanic populations. *Journal of Forensic
Sciences* 61 (5): 1311–1318.

Fowler, G. and Hughes, C. (2018). Development and assessment of postcranial sex estimation methods for a Guatemalan population. *Journal of Forensic Sciences* 63 (2): 490–496.

Garvin, H.M. and Passalacqua, N.V. (2012). Current practices by forensic anthropologists
in adult skeletal age estimation. *Journal of Forensic Sciences* 57 (2): 427–433.

Geller, P.L. (2009). Bodyscapes, biology, and heteronormativity. *American Anthropologist*
111 (4): 504–516.

Grivas, C.R. and Komar, D.A. (2008). Kumho, Daubert, and the nature of scientific
inquiry: implications for forensic anthropology. *Journal of Forensic Sciences* 53 (4):
771–776.

Hartnett, K.M. (2010). Analysis of age-at-death estimation using data from a new, modern
autopsy sample—part I: pubic bone. *Journal of Forensic Sciences* 55 (5): 1145–1151.

Jones, G. (2014). Not a yes or no question: critical perspectives on sex and gender in
forensic anthropology. MA thesis. University of Windsor.

Klales, A.R. (2016). Secular change in morphological pelvic traits used for sex estimation.
*Journal of Forensic Sciences* 61 (2): 295–301.

Kroman, A.M. and Symes, S.A. (2013). Investigation of skeletal trauma. In: *Research
Methods in Human Skeletal Biology* (ed. E.A. DiGangi and M.K. Moore), 219–239.
Waltham, MA: Elsevier.

Lesciotto, K.M. (2015). The impact of Daubert on the admissibility of forensic
anthropology expert testimony. *Journal of Forensic Sciences* 60 (3): 549–555.

Lewis, C.J. and Garvin, H.M. (2016). Reliability of the Walker cranial nonmetric method
and implications for sex estimation. *Journal of Forensic Sciences* 61 (3): 743–751.

Megyesi, M.S., Nawrocki, S.P., and Haskell, N.H. (2005). Using accumulated degree-days
to estimate the postmortem interval from decomposed human remains. *Journal of
Forensic Sciences* 50 (3): 1–9.

Parsons, H. R. (2017). The accuracy of the biological profile in casework: an analysis of
forensic anthropology reports in three medical examiner's offices. PhD thesis. University of Tennessee.

Santana, S.A., Bethard, J.D., and Moore, T.L. (2017). Accuracy of dental age in nonadults:
a comparison of two methods for age estimation using radiographs of developing teeth.
*Journal of Forensic Sciences* 62 (5): 1320–1325.

Steadman, D.W., Adams, B.J., and Konigsberg, L.W. (2006). Statistical basis for positive
identification in forensic anthropology. *American Journal of Physical Anthropology* 131
(1): 15–26.

Stewart, T.D. (1979). *Essentials of Forensic Anthropology: Especially as Developed in the United
States*. Springfield, IL: Charles C. Thomas.

Symes, S.A., L'Abbé, E.N., Stull, K.E. et al. (2014). Taphonomy and the timing of bone
fractures in trauma analysis. In: *Manual of Forensic Taphonomy* (ed. J.T. Pokines and S.A.
Symes), 341–365. Boca Raton, FL: CRC Press.

Tallman, S.D. and Go, M.C. (2018). Application of the optimized summed scored attributes method to sex estimation in Asian crania. *Journal of Forensic Sciences* 63 (3): 809–814.

Todd, T.W. (1920). Age changes in the pubic bone. I. The male white pubis. *American Journal of Physical Anthropology* 3 (3): 285–334.

## CHAPTER 4

# Expertise and the expert witness: contemporary educational foundations of forensic anthropology

Katelyn L. Bolhofner[1] and Andrew C. Seidel[2]

[1] *Texas Tech University, Lubbock, TX, USA*
[2] *Center for Bioarchaeological Research, School of Human Evolution and Social Change, Arizona State University, Tempe, AZ, USA*

"Every statement he made helped the case against the prisoner, *and yet it was abundantly evident that his sole concern was to present the exact truth as he knew it, exaggerating naught, and setting down naught in malice*. His voice was distinct and his exposition so clear that even the technical character of many of them did not prevent them from being understood by the jury. *His knowledge was so well systematized, so well in hand, so sound, precise, and broad, that it was a pleasure to listen to him*; it is not often one comes in contact with a brain of so fine fiber, so vigorous, and so sane" (Court Reporter Julian Hawthorne in reference to anthropologist George Dorsey; Hawthorne 1897).

The above is one of the earliest accounts of an anthropologist providing testimony within the United States judicial system. While this record of Dorsey's involvement in the Luetgert case remains an example to which all Forensic Anthropologists may aspire, it is but one highlight in the long history of anthropology in the courtroom – a story that includes the involvement of Harvard anatomists in the investigation of the murder of George Parkman in 1849, the regular cooperation between anthropologists at the Smithsonian and the FBI in the early twentieth century, and the eventual emergence of Forensic Anthropology as a distinct field of research in 1972. Regardless of the exact date or case, the work of an anthropologist as an expert witness often began with a box of bones dropped off at a university or museum by a police officer in need of aid. Asked to weigh in on the identity of the individual, to provide an opinion as to the post-mortem interval, or to offer an interpretation of traumatic injury evident in the skeletal remains, the physical anthropologist's expertise was called upon as a crucial component of a medico-legal investigation. This method for adopting casework led to the solidification of the discipline and, despite the increasing presence of Forensic Anthropologists working full-time within the medico-legal system, it remains a common occurrence today. Thus, the anthropologist is pulled into the workings of the justice system.

However, as Clyde Snow (1982, p. 101) so aptly pointed out, "the search for truth in the laboratory and the search for truth in the courtroom are games that are played by different rules." How, then, is an anthropologist to learn the rules of the courtroom? And how is the public, particularly members of a jury, to evaluate their work? How have standards of education and training changed over the past few decades, and what now qualifies an anthropologist to serve as an expert witness? How can the anthropologist be sure that their knowledge will be "systematized" and simultaneously "precise" and "broad," as Dorsey's was described? In this chapter, we will address these questions through a framework that examines the expertise of the Forensic Anthropologist as it has developed and evolved to meet new and changing expectations.

## 4.1   A brief historical overview of the discipline

In the United States, records of anatomists and anthropologists participating in medico-legal death investigations as experts extend to the mid nineteenth century. Famous murder investigations such as "The Parkman Murder" and "The Luetgert Case" enlisted experts such as Oliver Wendell Holmes, Jeffries Wyman, and George Dorsey to conduct identifications, trauma analyses, and to testify on behalf of the prosecution (Stewart 1978, 1979; Snow 1982). Following this slow beginning, Forensic Anthropology as a discipline began to take shape in the late 1930s, as academicians such as Wilton Krogman, T. Wingate Todd, T. Dale Stewart, Aleš Hrdlička, and Earnest Hooton provided intermittent services to law enforcement agencies during this time (Haviland 1994; Kerley 1978; Ubelaker 1999). In the 1940s, Krogman published a series of articles in the *FBI Law Enforcement Bulletin* that were circulated around the country (Krogman 1939, 1943; Krogman et al. 1948). These articles served to inform law enforcement agencies that experts were available to aid in skeletal identifications. During this time, the FBI began to regularly contact the anthropologists working at the Smithsonian for assistance in casework. Accompanying this increased reliance on the expertise of the anthropologist was a rise in published research related to identification and trauma in the recently deceased (e.g. Stewart 1948, 1951). But it was not until the 1960s and early 1970s that law enforcement regularly relied upon anthropologists to provide identifications in their investigations. Two seminal works, T. D.

Stewart's chapter on identification in Gradwohl's *Legal Medicine* (Stewart 1976) and Krogman's *The Human Skeleton in Forensic Medicine* (Krogman 1962), provided early "textbooks" on the subject as well as publicity regarding the utility of anthropologists to the medico-legal community. At this time, too, many coroner's offices that had been staffed with elected officials were replaced with medical examiner systems under the direction of forensic pathologists who increasingly sought out expert consultants to aid in medico-legal death investigations. The increase in physical anthropological research and its application in forensic contexts resulted in a number of important publications at this time (Bass 1969, 1979; Kerley 1978; İşcan 1988; Stewart 1976).

With the increased involvement of anthropologists in medico-legal contexts, education and training programs began to be offered that were tailored to methods in skeletal identification. Lawrence T. Angel began to offer an annual short course in skeletal identification for forensic pathologists and crime investigators at the Smithsonian Institution, and several academic institutions began programs to offer training and casework experience (Ubelaker 1997). Anthropologists working at the University of Kansas, the University of Tennessee, the University of Arizona, and the University of Florida provided coursework, mentorship, and casework opportunities to students beginning in the 1960s.

Despite this early work, the application of anthropology within the medico-legal system remained a relatively unorganized practice until, in the 1970s, a group of anthropologists who had regularly attended the American Academy of Forensic Sciences (AAFS) meeting in the General Section decided that anthropology should be recognized within the academy as a distinct discipline. As a result, the Physical Anthropology section (later revised to the Anthropology section) was created in 1972 (Kerley 1978; Snow 1982), an event often considered to mark the formal recognition of Forensic Anthropology as a field. This history has been described in detail in a number of volumes (e.g. Dirkmaat and Cabo 2012; Komar and Buikstra 2008), and its intricacies are outside the scope of this chapter. Here, in an effort to explore the origins of rigorous training, we instead focus upon the educational and experiential background of some of these founders of Forensic Anthropology, especially those individuals who laid the groundwork for expert testimony in the field.

## 4.2   The educational background of early forensic anthropologists

The major figures who paved the way for the formation of Forensic Anthropology as a field came from diverse backgrounds and educational programs, but with elements in common. A brief survey of their education and training provides a baseline for the standard of expertise to which Forensic Anthropologists should continue to look as basic elements necessary to qualify as an expert.

As noted previously, this historical overview is not meant to encompass all of the significant figures who contributed to the formation of the discipline. Rather, our focus in this chapter is to survey the educational backgrounds and training of those individuals who have lent their expertise to the witness stand and to examine the current state of these opportunities for students. As outlined in Table 4.1, the earliest expert witnesses in skeletal identification and trauma analysis had all achieved degrees at the highest level of their respective fields. Further, each had completed rigorous training in human anatomy, specifically in the context of medical training. Several of these individuals had also completed

**Table 4.1** Training, education, occupation, and the principle contributions of the earliest expert witnesses in skeletal identification and trauma analysis in the United States.

**Oliver Wendell Holmes, Sr. (1809–1894)**

| | |
|---|---|
| *Principle training* | *Principle occupation* |
| Physician, Poet | Private physician; Parkman Professor of Anatomy, Harvard College |
| *Highest degree attained* | *Principle contributions as an expert/expert witness* |
| MD | Expert for the prosecution in the Parkman Murder case |

**Jeffries Wyman (1814–1874)**

| | |
|---|---|
| *Principle training* | *Principle occupation* |
| Anatomist | Hersey Professor of Anatomy, Harvard College |
| *Highest degree attained* | *Principle contributions as an expert/expert witness* |
| MD | Testified for the prosecution in the Parkman Murder case |

**Thomas Dwight (1843–1911)**

| | |
|---|---|
| *Principle training* | *Principle occupation* |
| Physician, Anatomist | Parkman Professor of Anatomy, Harvard College |
| *Highest degree attained* | *Principle contributions as an expert/expert witness* |
| MD | "The Identification of the Human Skeleton: A Medicolegal Study" (1878) |

**Harris H. Wilder (1864–1928)**

| | |
|---|---|
| *Principle training* | *Principle occupation* |
| Zoologist, Anatomist | Smith College |
| *Highest degree attained* | *Principle contributions as an expert/expert witness* |
| PhD | "Personal Identification: Methods for the Identification of Individuals, Living or Dead" (1918) |

courses or had begun careers in law. Finally, these men all had some background in comparative vertebrate osteology and collaborated with pathologists, chemists, dentists, and other specialists in honing their knowledge and skill in preparing forensic reports. The education and knowledge of these early expert witnesses was truly both precise and broad.

If we look ahead to the founding of the Physical Anthropology section of the AAFS, we see this trend of diverse educational backgrounds, tied by a common thread of expertise in anatomy and skeletal biology, carried through. The founding members of the Physical Anthropology section of the AAFS included an MD, primatologists, and human biologists, but all members had some background in skeletal biology (see Komar and Buikstra 2008 for a thorough review). These members came to Forensic Anthropology from a variety of professional backgrounds and occupations, and only two of the founding members had developed dissertation research with direct forensic applications.

A survey of the educational background of the field of Forensic Anthropology provides a baseline for the expectation of expertise among practitioners in this field. However, only a few of these individuals spent significant time serving as expert witnesses. How is expertise translated and qualified so that one may serve as an expert witness? In Snow's terms, how does the education and training of an anthropologist apply within the rules of the courtroom game?

## 4.3   The forensic anthropologist as expert witness

An expert witness may be defined as an individual who offers a testimony based solely on an area of expertise. To be declared an expert witness, one must supply evidence of one's qualifications and/or certification in that field. A key difference between an expert witness and a material or fact witness is that the expert witness is allowed to offer an opinion based on their observations. The witness can be questioned regarding their training and qualifications by opposing counsel, but the ultimate decision to qualify an expert witness lies with the judge (see chapter 1 of Moenssens et al. 2017).

For the Forensic Anthropologist, being called to serve as an expert witness can occur in a number of ways. The full-time Forensic Anthropologist, employed in some capacity by the medico-legal system, often is called to testify based on their inclusion in the production of autopsy findings. The academician may be asked to analyze skeletal remains on a "public service" or "paid consultant" basis by either the law enforcement agency involved or by the defense counsel (see Chapter 12). According to the website of the American Board of Forensic Anthropology (ABFA), "once in court, Forensic Anthropologists view their role as educators. Their job is to try to teach the jury and others in the court about the basic principles that explain their scientific findings" (The American Board of Forensic Anthropology 2018). A quick Google search returns websites such as www.jurispro.com, which offers a list of "experts who may advise regarding Forensic Anthropology." Regardless of the manner in which the anthropologist is called to testify, their casework and academic training will be questioned during the qualification process. But what are the tenets by which Forensic Anthropologists may be qualified? What are the standards to which we should hold ourselves and our colleagues that they may be identified as "expert witnesses"?

To address these issues, in the 1970s, in cooperation with the AAFS and with a grant from the Law Enforcement Assistance Agency of the US Department of Justice, the Forensic Science Foundation provided funds for each section in the academy to develop a certification process (Snow 1982). In 1977, the Physical Anthropology section created the ABFA for the purpose of certifying Forensic Anthropologists in the United States. Modeled after the certification processes found within medical fields (Kerley 1978), the ABFA certification examination represents the culmination of forensic anthropological training, and requires that all examinees meet a number of academic and professional expectations and requirements (for current standards, see www.theabfa.org). Although their performance on individual cases is not guaranteed, anthropologists certified by the ABFA (referred to as Diplomates, or D-ABFAs) are considered by the profession to be qualified for participation in forensic casework (Komar and Buikstra 2008). Today, more than 40 years after the establishment of the ABFA, many anthropologists who testify in court remain uncertified. While this does not mean that such individuals lack the requisite education or experience, it is important to note that without achieving Diplomate status they are not recognized as meeting the national standards of practice within Forensic Anthropology. While ABFA certification is its apogee, the continuous process of training and education that characterizes the career of a contemporary Forensic Anthropologist is rooted in academic programs and institutes of higher education. With this in mind, the following section examines the typical structure and content of academic programs available to aspiring Forensic Anthropologists.

## 4.4   Current educational programs and training opportunities

In their 2008 volume, Komar and Buikstra noted the increased need for students of Forensic Anthropology to undergo rigorous, structured training in order to be prepared to testify as expert witnesses. Here, we explore the developments in such training programs in the decade since their call for increased rigor, noting those areas in which improvements should be made.

### 4.4.1  Contemporary educational programs for forensic anthropologists

Between its inception in 1977 and the time of this writing, the ABFA has certified 119 individuals as sufficiently qualified for involvement in forensic anthropological casework. Of these Board-certified Diplomates, 42 received their certification within the last decade and 27 only within the past five years. The period since 2012 has seen more individuals certified than at any time since the Board's formation (Figure 4.1). If such trends continue, a sizeable portion of the future population of D-ABFAs will have received their academic training in the educational programs of today. It is perhaps timely, then, to evaluate the academic programs available to aspiring Forensic Anthropologists in order to assess their strengths and weaknesses.

For inclusion in this review, an institution had to meet three criteria. The first criterion is that at least one D-ABFA, active or retired, must be listed as a faculty member within an academic department. The purpose of imposing this constraint is twofold. First, it counteracts the proliferation of programs that offer courses in Forensic Anthropology in an effort to capitalize on the popularity of television shows such as *Bones* or *CSI: Crime Scene Investigation*. Secondly, and more importantly, it ensures that instruction is at least potentially available from an individual who is already ABFA certified. The second criterion for inclusion in this review is that an institution must offer a graduate degree in either anthropology (regardless of whether a specialization in Forensic Anthropology is offered) or forensic sciences. As this chapter is a contribution to a book concerning the articulation between Forensic Anthropology and the United States judicial system, the third criterion is that an institution must be located within

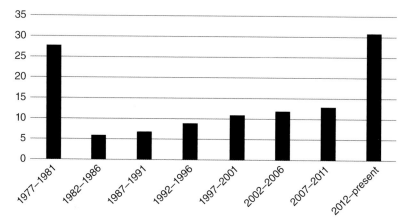

**Figure 4.1** Numbers of new Diplomates of the American Board of Forensic Anthropology through time.

**Table 4.2** Academic departments with D-ABFAs as faculty and degrees offered.

| DABFA departmental affiliation | n | Degrees offered |
|---|---|---|
| Anthropology | 23 | MA or MS in Anthropology, PhD in Anthropology (n=17) |
| Anatomy | 1 | MA in Forensic Anthropology, MS in Biomedical Forensic Sciences |
| Biology | 1 | MA or MS in Anthropology |
| Criminal Justice or Forensic Sciences | 2 | MS in Forensic Sciences, PhD in Forensic Sciences (n=1) |

the United States. Thus, while more than 40 academic institutions are fortunate enough to count one or more D-ABFAs among their faculty, the following characterization of contemporary graduate level educational programs for Forensic Anthropologists is based on a total of 27 different institutions. Table 4.2 presents the departmental affiliation of the Diplomates employed by these institutions as well as the degrees that they offer.

For each institution, a survey was made of all graduate-level coursework relevant to the practice of Forensic Anthropology offered within the past five years. In addition to courses dedicated specifically to Forensic Anthropology, the following six categories of courses were considered to be relevant: (i) biological or physical anthropology, (ii) bioarcheology or mortuary archeology, (iii) human osteology and/or skeletal biology, (iv) other forensic sciences, (v) human anatomy involving the dissection of cadavers, and (vi) criminal procedure and law. Although considerably more coarse-grained, these subject areas roughly parallel those included in an earlier survey of education within Forensic Anthropology (Galloway and Simmons 1997). The past five years of course catalogs for each institution were searched for graduate level coursework offered in the anthropology department. Where an anthropology department or institutional equivalent was nonexistent, the stated required curriculum and suggested electives for the graduate degree(s) offered were recorded. In addition, course catalogs for the past five years were searched for the following terms: "oste[ology]" and "skel[etal]" (in the event that coursework in human osteology was offered in a department other than anthropology), "forensic," "anatomy," "crim[inal]," and "legal." Where such catalogs were available online in searchable format, this was accomplished using a keyword search. In cases where archived catalogs were only available as downloadable PDF files, the full text was searched using the "Find" function in Adobe Acrobat Reader DC. For each institution, it was recorded whether or not graduate-level coursework was offered in Forensic Anthropology as well as each of the six categories listed above, and noted if such courses were available within academic departments outside of that with which a D-ABFA was affiliated. As it is not the intention of this chapter to criticize or praise any particular academic institution(s), these results were then aggregated in order to illustrate trends in the formal education currently available to students of Forensic Anthropology and compared with the coursework available within the subset of institutions offering a PhD in anthropology, as this is a prerequisite for ABFA certification (Figure 4.2).

Graduate-level courses with Forensic Anthropology as their primary topic are only offered by 59.3% of the institutions in the study sample, a proportion that decreases to 47.1% of those institutions that offer a doctoral degree in anthropology. Graduate coursework in biological or physical anthropology exhibits a trend in the opposite direction, increasing from being offered in 77.8% of all institutions under consideration to being available in 88.2% of institutions offering a PhD. In general, however, the majority of academic departments with Diplomates as faculty members offer graduate level coursework in both biological or physical anthropology and human osteology and/or skeletal anatomy, while approximately half of such departments offer graduate courses whose specific foci include Forensic Anthropology, bioarcheology, or mortuary analysis. While the observed emphasis on physical anthropology and human osteology is unsurprising given that the vast majority of D-ABFAs are trained as physical anthropologists and/or skeletal biologists, the relative rarity of courses focusing on Forensic Anthropology or bioarcheology is somewhat unexpected.

Of more immediate concern, however, is the near absence of intradepartmental graduate coursework pertaining to other forensic sciences, as well as to criminal procedure and law. Among institutions offering doctoral degrees in anthropology, such coursework is only available within academic departments distinct from those that include D-ABFAs among their faculty, and often are only offered by institutionally affiliated law schools. The result is that formal education in these aspects of Forensic Anthropology is largely unavailable to students. This is not to say that students are not exposed to the medico-legal side of Forensic Anthropology – many courses that provide an overview of the discipline include discussion of topics such as the medico-legal and judicial systems, as well as crime scene investigation and expert witness testimony. Rather, it is to suggest that the educational training of Forensic Anthropologists is decidedly uneven. For a discipline that applies the theories and techniques of physical anthropology within a medico-legal context, contemporary educational programs for Forensic Anthropologists provide much more training regarding osteological and anthropological techniques than knowledge of the context in which such techniques will be applied.

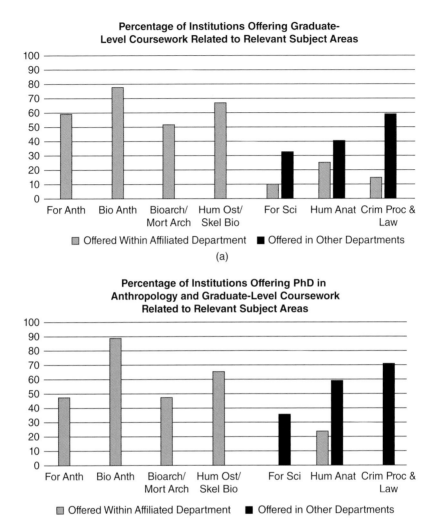

**Figure 4.2** A comparison of the kinds of graduate coursework offered that is relevant to Forensic Anthropology in (a) all institutions in the current sample and (b) the 17 institutions that offer a PhD in anthropology.

There are several limitations to the characterization of graduate education for Forensic Anthropologists provided above. First, decisions made as to whether or not a given course and its content is relevant to Forensic Anthropology are inherently subjective. Such decisions were made based on our own educational experiences, as well as topics that we have found to be relevant in our extra-curricular training and involvement with forensic anthropological casework. The associations between the subject areas considered here and the practice of Forensic Anthropology, however, are lent some validity by their broad similarity to topics considered in an earlier, more nuanced review of education in Forensic Anthropology (Galloway and Simmons 1997). Secondly, this review is coarse-grained, relying on course titles and descriptions for its data and emphasizing the primary foci of available coursework. For example, although human osteology may be included as a component of a graduate-level overview of Forensic Anthropology, a given institution was only considered to offer graduate coursework in this topic if one or more courses emphasizing human osteology were available at the graduate level. This approach also excluded those institutions for which human osteology was offered only at the undergraduate level. Lastly, this review only considered those institutions at which one or more faculty members are D-ABFAs, resulting in a relatively small sample size. As stated above, this constraint was employed in order to guarantee at least the potential for training under the supervision and mentorship of a Board-certified Forensic Anthropologist. This choice perhaps reflects the bias of the authors, for whom such training has proved to not only be invaluable, but as we will argue in the following section, it also reflects the purpose of the creation of the ABFA. Without training and mentorship toward certification, the field will continue to suffer from a lack of regulatory oversight (Christensen and Crowder 2009).

### 4.4.2 Casework and training opportunities

Beyond the required educational background, we argue here that casework and training opportunities should be an integral component in building the expertise of a Forensic Anthropologist. Yet this type of hands-on experience is not explicitly offered or required by most educational programs surveyed. Instead, the model observed in most graduate-level institutions where a D-ABFA is affiliated is one of internship or informal mentorship. Alternatively, a student of Forensic Anthropology could seek out additional training in short, hands-on courses or field schools offered by a number of colleges and universities. Here, we review several of those opportunities and models.

Hands-on training in skeletal anatomy and trauma analysis are central to the development of expertise in Forensic Anthropology. Several universities in the United States offer short courses and internships in various forensic techniques that provide hands-on experience for advanced undergraduate and graduate students. For example, in addition to a variety of short courses focusing on forensic anthropological field and laboratory work, the University of Tennessee Knoxville's Forensic Anthropology Center offers a summer internship that provides experience in the processing of skeletal remains through a mock forensic case. Similarly, the Forensic Anthropology Center at Texas State also offers a summer internship providing experience in the processing of skeletal remains, as well as the potential for advanced students to assist in forensic archeological work. Mercyhurst University also offers summer short courses in topics such as death investigation, biological profile construction, and trauma analysis. While these short courses offer valuable training to students, they often do not entail participation in active casework.

Fellowship in the AAFS and certification by the ABFA are recognized in the legal system as important aspects of the scientific qualification of expert witnesses. In order to become certified, an individual must have completed their PhD in anthropology or a related field, and they must demonstrate practical experience in the form of completed case reports. While certification is not required to perform casework or to testify in court, it offers a measure by which the expertise of the anthropologist can be assessed, and therefore we argue that it should become a standard expectation in the education and training of Forensic Anthropologists. But if casework is not a typical component of the training in educational programs or internships, how does one obtain the casework experience necessary to qualify to take the board examination?

At its inception, the board certification process outlined by the ABFA was meant to provide a three-year period in which postdoctoral casework could be completed in preparation for the exam and status as a Diplomate. As the field has evolved and become more visible in the medico-legal system, however, Diplomate status is often a prerequisite for casework in medical examiner systems and for consultations with lawyers and investigators, thus opportunities for a postdoctoral, pre-certification anthropologist to participate in casework during this period can be limited. Further complicating this process, the increased opportunities for graduate students to participate in casework prior to this official three-year period, but an inability to sit for the examination until this period of waiting has ended, leaves a number of newly minted professionals without the certification necessary to move forward with their careers. In light of these complications, the ABFA voted in 2018 to move forward with the restructuring of these prerequisites. In the future, more weight will be given to evaluating an individual's casework and training in assessing their qualification to sit for the exam, regardless of whether the experience was gained during graduate or postdoctoral work.

Despite these changes, currently there are limited formal channels providing opportunities for graduate students – or even postdoctoral individuals – to participate in active casework. Several graduate institutions do offer students the opportunity to participate in active casework under the oversight of a D-ABFA. Others offer the promise of graduate student participation through existing laboratory/medical examiner office relationships, but without the ensured oversight and mentorship of a D-ABFA we cannot recommend such avenues. Additionally, these casework opportunities may not offer comprehensive exposure to both biological profile and trauma assessment. However, as we have outlined in the previous section, the pursuit of a graduate degree under the advisement of a D-ABFA, or at an institution with which a D-ABFA is actively associated, should provide the mentorship necessary to gain experience in casework. Alternatively, a qualified graduate student in a skeletal biology, anthropology, or related discipline and without access to direct mentorship is encouraged to contact a D-ABFA with whom they are interested in working to inquire as to the potential for establishing a mentoring relationship.

## 4.5   Conclusion and future directions

In his "An 'outsider' look at forensic anthropology," James Adovasio writes that, "even a casual perusal of the literature of Forensic Anthropology from the past several decades reveals that there is little general agreement, and perhaps even none, concerning the fundamental nature of this field" (Adovasio 2012). Even if one does not particularly agree with this assessment, they are still left with the reality that beyond a PhD there currently is no standard in education or training expected of Forensic Anthropologists offering their expertise as expert witnesses. When offering scientific evidence in civil and criminal cases, the anthropologist must justify their personal education, experience, and the peer-reviewed, academic nature of the methods used in their assessments. This complex interaction between the Forensic Anthropologist and the legal system is the focus of this volume as a whole and beyond the scope of this chapter. Here, we have presented the educational foundations of the field and the current state of educational and training opportunities in the United States. In this final section, we offer a few lessons from this review in the hope that future outsiders will look to our field and see a "fundamental nature" that is characterized by established standards of education and training.

In his 1982 review of the state of the field, Clyde Snow argued that it would be "unwise to permit students to specialize in Forensic Anthropology at the expense of more traditional areas of anthropological knowledge" (p. 113). Similarly, if there is a lesson to be learned from an examination of the educational foundations of Forensic Anthropologists who served as expert witnesses, it is perhaps that educational programs for Forensic Anthropology can be improved by requiring increased diversity through the implementation of courses in anatomy and law. In particular, we argue that cadaver-based courses should become a standard expectation of education in human anatomy. While 64.7% of institutions offering PhDs in anthropology offer graduate coursework in human osteology, only 23.5% of such institutions offer intradepartmental courses in human anatomy. An in-depth understanding of the articulation of hard tissue and soft tissue is extremely useful in the interpretation of skeletal remains, especially in those cases involving trauma analysis. As illustrated in Figure 4.2, contemporary educational programs offering degrees in anthropology do not typically require (and may not even offer) graduate coursework in these subject areas.

Further, curricula that cross disciplinary boundaries to incorporate training in criminal and legal procedures, including evidence processing and crime scene protocol, would greatly facilitate the translation of expertise into efficacy as an expert witness. The institutional infrastructure for providing graduate coursework in criminal procedure and law already exists in many cases, as evidenced by the observation that 70.6% of institutions offering doctorate degrees in anthropology offer such courses in other departments (Figure 4.2b). Courses emphasizing medico-legal death investigation, criminal procedure and law, evidence, and expert witness testimony potentially could be developed through inter-departmental collaborations. Of particular utility for students of Forensic Anthropology would be courses that take the format of a mock trial, in which students are required to provide expert testimony and are critiqued by their peers. Such courses are already offered by some institutions offering master's degrees in Forensic Anthropology, but seemingly remain absent from those offering doctoral degrees.

With the changing shape of the field, particularly the increased expectation that practicing and aspiring Forensic Anthropologists become ABFA certified, efforts should be made to offer opportunities for hands-on training and casework experience as standard components of education in this field. Whether this training takes the form of short courses, mentorships, internships, or as a component of graduate coursework, the student of Forensic Anthropology must have the opportunity to gain this experience.

Finally, engagement in forensic casework under the supervision of a D-ABFA will encourage participation in the ABFA certification process and help to ensure that national standards of training and education are being met. Such standardization is important for the involvement of Forensic Anthropologists within the judicial system, as it will help to minimize the subjectivity introduced into analyses as a result of differing levels of experience. While this type of mentorship is a costly commitment on the part of the D-ABFA, who is often working full-time in a medico-legal context or attempting to balance casework with academic responsibilities and research, the potential benefit to the field of Forensic Anthropology as a whole is immeasurable. Until the imbalance between "forensic" and "anthropology" within contemporary academic programs is resolved, the experiences of those anthropologists who have served as expert witnesses will remain one of the best sources of information for those practitioners who find themselves called to testify for the first time.

# References

Adovasio, J.M. (2012). An "outsider" look at forensic anthropology. In: *A Companion to Forensic Anthropology* (ed. D.C. Dirkmaat), 683–689. Hoboken, NJ: Blackwell Publishing Ltd.

Bass, W.M. (1969). Recent developments in the identification of human skeletal material. *American Journal of Physical Anthropology* 30: 459–461.

Bass, W.M. (1979). Developments in the identification of human skeletal material (1968-1978). *American Journal of Physical Anthropology* 51: 555–562.

Christensen, A.M. and Crowder, C.M. (2009). Evidentiary standards for forensic anthropology. *Journal of Forensic Sciences* 54 (6): 1211–1216.

Dirkmaat, D.C. and Cabo, L.L. (2012). Forensic anthropology: embracing the new paradigm. In: *A Companion to Forensic Anthropology* (ed. D.C. Dirkmaat), 3–40. Hoboken, NJ: Blackwell Publishing Ltd.

Galloway, A. and Simmons, T.L. (1997). Education in forensic anthropology: appraisal and outlook. *Journal of Forensic Sciences* 42: 796–801.

Haviland, W.A. (1994). Wilton Marion Krogman. *National Academy of Sciences. Biographical Memoirs* 63: 292–321.

Hawthorne, J. (1897), The Luetgert Trial. *The Chicago Tribune* (17 September).

Iscan, M.Y. (1988). Rise of forensic anthropology. *Yearbook of Physical Anthropology* 31: 203–230.

Kerley, E.R. (1978). Recent developments in forensic anthropology. *Yearbook of Physical Anthropology* 21: 160–173.

Komar, D.A. and Buikstra, J.E. (2008). *Forensic Anthropology: Contemporary Theory and Practice*. New York: Oxford University Press.

Krogman, W.M. (1939). A guide to the identification of human skeletal material. *FBI Law Enforcement Bulletin* 8 (8): 3–31.

Krogman, W.M. (1943). Role of the physical anthropologist in the identification of human skeletal remains. *FBI Law Enforcement Bulletin* 12 (4): 17, 12(5), 12–40, 28.

Krogman, W.M. (1962). *The Human Skeleton in Forensic Medicine*. Springfield, IL: Charles C. Thomas.

Krogman, W.M., McGregor, J., and Frost, B. (1948). A problem in human skeletal remains. *FBI Law Enforcement Bulletin* 17 (6): 7–12.

Moenssens, A.A., DesPortes, B.L., and Benjamin, S.D. (eds.) (2017). Scientific evidence and expert testimony. In: *Scientific Evidence in Civil and Criminal Cases*, 7e. St. Paul: Foundation Press.

Snow, C.C. (1982). Forensic anthropology. *Annual Review of Anthropology* 11: 97–131.

Stewart, T.D. (1948). Medicolegal aspects of the skeleton, I. Sex, age, race, and stature. *American Journal of Physical Anthropology* 6: 135–322.

Stewart, T.D. (1951). What the bones tell. *FBI Law Enforcement Bulletin* 20 (2): 2–5, 19.

Stewart, T.D. (1976). Identification by skeletal structures. In: *Gradwohl's Legal Medicine*, 3e, 109–135. Bristol: Francis E. Camps.

Stewart, T.D. (1978). George A. Dorsey's role in the Luetgert case: a significant episode in the history of forensic anthropology. *Journal of Forensic Sciences* 23 (4): 786–791.

Stewart, T.D. (1979). *Essentials of Forensic Anthropology*. Springfield, IL: Charles C. Thomas.

The American Board of Forensic Anthropology. (2018). Frequently Asked Questions. http://theabfa.org/faq/students/ (accessed October 19, 2018).

Ubelaker, D.H. (1997). Forensic anthropology. In: *History of Physical Anthropology: An Encyclopedia*, vol. 1 (ed. F. Spenser), 392–396. New York: Garland Publishing.

Ubelaker, D.H. (1999). Aleš Hrdlička's role in the history of forensic anthropology. *Journal of Forensic Sciences* 44 (4): 724–730.

**PART II**
# The rubber meets the road

**CHAPTER 5**

# Transparency in forensic anthropology through the implementation of quality assurance practices

Julie M. Fleischman[1], Michal L. Pierce[1], and Christian M. Crowder[2]

[1] *Harris County Institute of Forensic Sciences, Houston, TX, USA*
[2] *Southwestern Institute of Forensic Sciences, Dallas, TX, USA*

## 5.1   Introduction

The quest for transparency in the forensic sciences is guided by robust quality assurance (QA) programs; however, antiquated ideas of what QA is and how it is applied is a roadblock for many laboratories. First, all forensic disciplines must abandon the "old school" thinking that QA only pertains to the hard sciences and therefore exists exclusively in the crime laboratory. This is a fallacy. All fields need and benefit from QA. We must now see modern QA for what it is today – a positive, proactive way of thinking, instead of a simple means for rigidly defining conformity. Secondly, the forensic disciplines must recognize the difference between quality control (QC, QA), and quality management (QM). QC focuses on testing the conformity of a product or service, while QA ensures that processes are conducive for generating a quality product or service. QM is broader and involves the planning and policy-making of top management to support QC, QA, and quality improvement initiatives.

In a laboratory setting, the product is usually a report of analytical findings. Alternatively, if a formal report will not be issued, the resulting service is either a verbal consult for opinion or perhaps expert testimony. These products or services must meet a level of quality deemed acceptable to the customer. While the terms "customer," "provider," and "product" may seem odd to forensic scientists, particularly anthropologists who do not tend to think of their work in this manner, these terms are used in the QM vernacular. From a quality perspective, a customer is defined as the individual/group who will receive the finished product (i.e. forensic pathologist, law enforcement officer, attorneys, etc.),

*Forensic Anthropology and the United States Judicial System*, First Edition.
Edited by Laura C. Fulginiti, Kristen Hartnett-McCann, and Alison Galloway.
© 2019 John Wiley & Sons Ltd. Published 2019 by John Wiley & Sons Ltd.

while the provider is the forensic scientist or laboratory conducting the analysis. Different customers view quality differently. Some feel that a quality service means the product is free from technical errors. Others, depending on the location or setting of the workplace, define quality as adherence to predefined requirements or standards. The various requirements may come internally (i.e. employer directives or management system), from the customers themselves, or an external source (e.g. accrediting body or legal statutes). Yet another definition of quality is the ability to cater to the customer's needs, both the stated and implied. Once the quality requirements are established (it can be a combination of the above three options), the provider can begin to plan their program for managing, assessing, and, eventually improving the quality of their work.

The most common model for improving quality is that of the Plan-Do-Check-Act (PDCA) cycle. Invented by Dr. Walter A. Shewhart in 1939 (Shewhart 1939), and modified by Dr. W. Edwards Deming for the Japanese in 1950 (Deming 1950), this model has remained relevant for decades in every type of industry. The concept behind PDCA is as follows: (i) plan the intended change by deciding what actions are needed to achieve the change; (ii) perform the actions to carry out the change, either in a pilot program or on a small scale; (iii) assess the results and effectiveness of the changes; and (iv) proceed accordingly. That is, if the change led to unintended consequences, determine their cause and go back to step (i) to modify the plan. If the change was deemed successful, then fully implement and incorporate the change into the standard operating procedure (SOP). The model's simplicity is what makes it applicable to any business size and type. The "plan" portion reminds us that quality must always be a planned activity – if an unplanned event was successful, it was just luck. The "check" and "act" portions remind us of the importance of measuring, assessing, and adjusting operations as appropriate. Like all good science, our conclusions, and therefore required actions, should be based on observations and data. The PDCA cycle can be used not only to implement desired improvements, but also to fix problems (i.e. corrective action).

The PDCA cycle, along with other quality models not mentioned here, are based on systematic and objective approaches which are equally applicable to disciplines that lend themselves to more subjective interpretations, such as anthropology and pathology. Therefore, a quality program ensures that forensic providers/services conduct their examinations systematically and objectively. Should a case be litigated, or if the anthropologist is required to provide expert testimony, having quality procedures in place lends validity and support to the scientific analysis. For example, while an expert is expected to testify about their findings with unwavering confidence, what assurances does the jury have that the anthropologist is proficient at what they do, or that the case has been handled systematically and objectively? Or that the anthropologist offers an opinion with which another, similarly qualified anthropologist would concur? If the answer to any of these questions is "because the expert said so," then that is the wrong answer. Although members of the jury may still be inclined to accept an expert's opinion at face value simply because the expert possesses a PhD, the role of judges as gatekeepers should ensure that there is sufficient scientific evidence and methodology to support the expert's opinion. Furthermore, effective counsel will not permit an expert to testify simply because the expert is well educated. The doctoral degree and years of experience are significant qualifiers for the examiner, but what speaks for the examination itself? A few QA measures, at a minimum, or a comprehensive QA program, will demonstrate that the examination has been conducted under established guidelines and bolsters the surety, and thus the admissibility, of the anthropological report.

As stated earlier, aspiring to be as error-free as possible and adhering to specific predetermined requirements demonstrates a desire to produce quality work. However, the QA program is what sets the anthropologist on the path to achieve this, and, if executed correctly with the application of valid scientific methods, will yield documented proof that quality measures were carried out. Whether or not the QA records are physically brought to court, being able to discuss them on the stand will make a significant impact on the reliability and weight of one's testimony. Merely speaking about the quality concepts and practices employed within the laboratory can demonstrate professional responsibility, and a commitment to best practices within the field. This addition can also assist in refuting arguments that your report or opinion is a product of "junk science." The practitioner can arm themselves with measures to ensure that they are delivering a quality service with documented training, validated methods, established procedures, peer reviewed case records, calibrated equipment, secured information databases, protected evidence handling areas, and continued proficiency.

When claiming that the work performed is reliable and of high quality, the laboratory personnel are certifying that any analyses were carried out objectively, with all concerted efforts to be as unbiased as possible. This holds true even for more subjective anthropological analyses (e.g. developing an age-at-death interval from multiple methods/elements, morphoscopic ancestry estimation, etc.). While the level of subjectivity may vary depending on the methods employed or the amount of interpretation required, having a QA program indicates that the procedures to examine remains and collect data are transparent and systematic. The underlying concept of QA is that, even in a laboratory of one, an equally qualified examiner can review the laboratory's protocols to check for adherence either to specific program standards or generally accepted practices within the field. In fact, when such a review does take place, the laboratory's quality program can be bolstered if the reviewer offers suggestions for improvement. Frequently, an outside, unbiased perspective can greatly assist management with identifying potentially weaker or outdated areas of an operation, even when nothing is definitively wrong.

## 5.2 Overview of laboratory quality assurance and management

### 5.2.1 Corrective and preventive actions

Transparency and accountability are end results of a good QA program, and are also important within the judicial process. Although good QM focuses on service improvements and preventing problems from occurring (i.e. preventive actions), the reality is that problems and nonconformities do occur. How a practitioner chooses to handle nonconforming work or an identified mistake speaks to the level of quality within that laboratory.

A strong QA program will include a procedure for investigating identified errors to perform a root cause analysis. Once the root cause of an error is determined, ideas for mitigating or eliminating the cause should be developed; this is followed by a single chosen course of action to provide the most effective outcome. Herein lies the beginning of the PDCA cycle. The four steps of PDCA are then followed to implement the change that will ensure the same mistake is not repeated within the laboratory. This process allows for a sense of accountability on the part of the laboratory or practitioner. Although it is impossible to reverse the offending action, moving forward with the intent to better oneself, for the sake of the field, demonstrates a sense of professional responsibility that the public can appreciate.

While seemingly counterintuitive to speak about problems, mistakes, or corrective actions on the stand for fear of being seen as less of an expert, or less intelligent, in the current judicial climate, transparency is not only encouraged for a forensic service provider, it is expected. This means that any issues or mistakes discovered during or after a forensic analysis should be appropriately documented and available for discovery, and even disclosed during testimony. A QA program will therefore include a procedure for documenting nonconforming work within the casefile, including how to maintain any applicable corrective action records, as well as a policy for disclosing errors to any stakeholder of the case. The ability to speak openly to the jury or judge about an unintentional error that may have occurred, what impact it had on the case (if any), and what measures were taken to correct and ensure it will not happen in the future, communicates a level of accountability and professionalism that they can trust.

## 5.3 Training and continuous education

Traditionally, training has been viewed as a separate activity from QA or QM. This is particularly true for the education of most Forensic Anthropologists. The ability to independently analyze forensic evidence is typically acquired through coursework/fieldwork experience during graduate school, and then followed by shadowing a mentor post degree. With the exception of a few universities with well-established Forensic Anthropology laboratories, the concept of QA is not typically incorporated into this academic-level training and education. However, good training is the key to building a solid foundation for a competent practitioner. Therefore, an effective training program should include QA; and a laboratory's QA program should incorporate training. Quality forensic services are most effectively delivered when best practices, professional ethics, and the concepts regarding SOPs are learned during the formative years of training.

Good training and mentoring will lead to competent practitioners, however, some laboratories or practitioners may be unaware of this fact if they have never conducted a root cause analysis of nonconforming work. For example, if a problem is identified in an employee's work, the employee's supervisor or designee needs to determine what caused the error or departure from acceptable practice. When this is a first-time offense, the root cause is frequently attributed to the employee having never been informed of or shown the proper protocol. Or, if the employee was aware of the protocol, perhaps it was not demonstrated effectively. In other words, the employee was not trained properly. After retraining the employee in the specific task or protocol, rather than reprimanding the employee – as is common in this type of scenario – a more effective strategy is to check whether other employees have an adequate grasp on the protocol, and act accordingly. If the problem was limited to the one employee, this should be noted for future hires, and the training or orientation for new hires should be modified to prevent the same occurrence. If the problem is more systemic (meaning others could have potentially made the same mistake), then remedial training is necessary for all laboratory employees, not just the one individual who was "caught."

Forensic laboratories should develop a training program for all employees. The training program should consist of two tracks: one track for less experienced practitioners (e.g. recent graduates, new hires with limited hands-on training, or those who have not conducted independent analyses), and another track for experienced practitioners (i.e. those who were qualified as independent examiners in their previous place of employment). After both the inexperienced and experienced examiners receive training on agency policies, protocols, and office/laboratory culture – which should not be skipped, as these are vital components of QM – the two training tracks will diverge. The less experienced practitioners will undergo a period of training and supervision to learn about the concepts and methods generally employed in the laboratory until the supervisor deems the trainee capable enough to practice independently. One or more competency exams could be issued to the trainee to assist with this determination. For the experienced practitioner, the recommendation is that they should read the department's policies and SOPs and take a competency exam. If the practitioner passes the exam, they are immediately authorized to commence independent casework, with periodic administrative guidance as necessary. If the competency exam indicates the practitioner is not yet ready for independent casework, a period of abbreviated training or supervision should be required to address the area(s) requiring attention. This should not be seen as punishment for the new hire; it simply indicates that training in a prior laboratory was insufficient or different. This type of training, before commencing independent casework, will prevent serious errors from occurring in the future.

The final piece of the training program, which should be provided to both the less and more experienced practitioners, is continuing education and professional development. All practitioners should be committed to lifelong learning within their field, which includes staying abreast of new methods, new technologies, and significant discussions in the literature. The concept of continuous education is therefore a significant component of improving the quality of work. Equally important, honing one's skills in communication, time management, and expert testimony effectively serves the customer, which is why anthropologists should periodically seek professional development courses or opportunities to further exercise these administrative skills.

## 5.4   Importance of QA for anthropologists

Implementation of a QA program is more challenging in forensic anthropology compared with other forensic disciplines, such as toxicology and genetics. The latter disciplines have more technical equipment and automated processes, which are easier to regulate and control within a laboratory setting. Forensic Anthropologists, however, must contend with the ultimate nonstandardized data: human variation. Characterizing and evaluating human variation often lends itself to more subjective methods. Thus, the challenges associated with qualifying and quantifying human variation set anthropology apart from the other hard sciences. A robust quality program provides a layer of checks and controls to assist with the standardization of procedures.

The importance of QA for forensic anthropology practitioners is evident even beyond the laboratory. For example, what happens when a Forensic Anthropologist is on the stand as an expert witness? The *voir dire* process establishes the anthropologist as an expert in the field (i.e. questions regarding educational background, certifications held, employment history, experience, etc.). While the anthropologist has demonstrated that they are adequately qualified within the field of forensic anthropology, what criteria have qualified them to perform work on this particular case, for this particular agency?

In a laboratory with multiple practitioners or, at the very least, an involved administrative supervisor, qualification may be demonstrated by the completion of a documented training program. A practitioner who can provide the court with supporting documentation, such as a memorandum of authorization for independent casework from a supervisor, or information regarding the completion of a competency exam with a passing grade (the American Board of Forensic Anthropology (ABFA) exam is one example), is a practitioner who establishes that they were properly trained and are competent to perform the analyses in question. In addition to becoming a Diplomate by passing the ABFA exam, which certifies that you possess the core skills/foundations to be a practitioner, proficiency exams within your laboratory should (if available) be completed to demonstrate the degree of continued aptitude. For single practitioners/contractors, the concept behind a documented training program is still achievable. Devise a training program that can be implemented in the event that you acquire an intern or a fellow, or perhaps have the opportunity to expand your service to include associates. Demonstrating the ability to develop such a program will highlight the value you place on proper training, and therefore, your quality as a practitioner. It will position you as the authority on how to perform quality forensic anthropological service in your organization, and show that you have considered the important elements of your management system that make a competent, functional practitioner.

## 5.5 Quality assurance for forensic anthropology methods and equipment

### 5.5.1 Establishing laboratory SOPs

All Forensic Anthropology laboratories – whether in an academic institution, medical examiner's office, post-conflict zone, or military institution – must have SOPs that guide analyses and the handling of equipment and evidence. A procedure is defined as a "specified way to carry out an activity or a process" (ISO/IEC 17000 2004). The goals of an SOP are to inform staff regarding the proper way to carry out a task, and to establish a minimum level of uniformity among the staff when carrying out the same activity. While most forensic accreditation programs do not mandate specific elements or formats for SOPs, they should include the following elements for clarity: purpose, intent, procedures, references (if applicable), the name or position title of the owner of the document, and revision date(s). Ultimately, agencies and laboratories have leeway to write and standardize their own procedures to best accommodate their activities and customers.

As general guidance an SOP should accommodate the most "normal" or "typical" situation encountered in the laboratory; there will always be exceptions, but the document should be written so that it can be followed without frequent deviations.

Accrediting bodies do, however, require the presence of SOPs addressing administration, technical, and quality procedures to ensure effective laboratory operations. The absence of these procedures will jeopardize the effectiveness and quality of the laboratory's operations and lead to errors that would otherwise be avoidable. Here are examples of SOPs addressing the three required categories mentioned above: (i) Administration: hiring, training, evaluating personnel, and information safeguarding; (ii) Technical: evidence (i.e. identification, collection, handling, packaging, transport, and disposition), examination, validation or verification of methods, technical/peer review, and guidelines for interpretation and reporting; and (iii) Quality: control of documents, control of records, equipment maintenance, instrument calibration, internal audits, corrective action, preventive action, safety precautions, and any necessary QC of testing. Depending upon the services provided by your laboratory and the number of Forensic Anthropologists or staff, some of these procedures may not apply. Each laboratory must assess the types of procedures they need and standardize them accordingly to avoid errors and inefficiency.

An SOP should undergo an independent review once it has been written by the Forensic Anthropologist(s). In an ideal context, this review would be performed by a QA representative or an individual specifically trained in QA and QC. While this may not always be possible, particularly in academic institutions or single-practitioner laboratories, having a designated QA specialist – or at the very least, an external Forensic Anthropologist – to review SOPs provides a non-biased assessment of the procedure.

From the perspective of the authors' Quality Management Division, the review of SOPs assesses compliance with accreditation standards and/or the rest of the agency's policies and management procedures. In other words, a new or revised SOP should not contradict another procedure/policy or violate any accreditation requirements. Although the QA reviewer may be less familiar with the anthropological administration, techniques, or equipment being described in the SOP, this individual may spot gaps in the procedure or provide suggestions for additional elements that can be added for further clarity. The SOP should be specific enough to adequately instruct staff and prevent them from making errors, but general enough to allow for flexibility – writing an overly specific SOP results in frequent deviations from the procedure, which indicates a poorly written procedure. Ultimately the QA review ensures that any anthropologist entering the laboratory (i.e. new hires, interns, visiting scientists/researchers, etc.) will be able to read the SOP, and in conjunction with training, implement the methods or use the equipment effectively.

Once the SOP is approved by the author(s) and reviewed by the QA representative it is ready for distribution and implementation in the laboratory. Each anthropologist working in the laboratory will read the new SOP to become familiar with the method, process, or equipment being implemented, and will practice the new or revised technique(s). To demonstrate comprehension of the SOP and the ability to perform the procedure independently, a competency test – written by either the manager, QA representative, or an external Forensic Anthropologist – is administered. As mentioned above, a passing grade on the competency test provides documentation (for auditors, managers/supervisors, professors, laboratory directors, judges/juries, etc.) that the anthropologist has read and adequately understands the SOP and the method, technique, or equipment being used. This documentation of competency is vital should the anthropologists' training, analyses, or interpretations be called into question in a judicial setting.

Competency is then "spot checked" over subsequent months and years through proficiency testing. A proficiency test is given to staff at regular, planned intervals to ensure continued competence (i.e. skills or knowledge are being maintained). Proficiency tests may evaluate practitioner error and identify knowledge gaps that can be resolved with additional training. At the authors' workplace the Quality Management Division administers at least one proficiency test each year for the Forensic Anthropologists. The specific procedures/skills tested (i.e. ancestry estimation, human/non-human assessment, age-at-death estimation, etc.) alternate each year. For example, the Forensic Anthropology Division (FAD) at the Harris County Institute of Forensic Sciences (HCIFS) wrote a new craniometrics SOP, specifically addressing the collection of craniometric data using the MicroScribe three-dimensional digitizer and its associated software (i.e. 3Skull and Advantage Data Architect). After the anthropologists read the new SOP, were trained to properly use the digitizer and software, and were observed by the FAD Director, a competency test was administered to document each anthropologist's ability to use the equipment to perform independent casework. Now that competency has been achieved by all of the anthropologists, craniometric data collection can be added to the rotation of future proficiency testing for the FAD staff.

## 5.6  Various measures of quality

The question is, why should well-established anthropological methods that have been published in peer reviewed journals, and equipment that is already accepted in the scholarly community be validated? Perhaps the methods and/or equipment do work well and are valid in the field at-large (Pierce et al. 2016), but the crucial element for QA is *internal* validation and verification. Each Forensic Anthropology laboratory needs to demonstrate that the methods and equipment being used are working properly in their laboratory, and that personnel are properly trained and qualified to use such methods and equipment. This internal testing and documentation provides accountability and transparency indicating that you have critically assessed your methods, procedures, equipment, and staff.

All accredited laboratories, or any laboratory striving for higher standards of operation, must review significant factors that may contribute to error, variability, or decreased quality of their analytical outputs. There are various measures of quality and steps that can be taken to ensure analytical reliability; those most applicable to Forensic Anthropology laboratories are calibration, validation/verification, proficiency testing (described above), and establishing error and uncertainty of measurement.

Calibration is defined by the International Bureau of Weights and Measures (*Bureau International des Poids et Mesures*, BIPM) as a set of operations that establish, under specified conditions, the relationship between values of quantities indicated by a measuring instrument or measuring system, or values represented by a material measure or a reference material, and the corresponding values realized by the standards (Joint Committee for Guides in Metrology 2008b). What follows is a non-exhaustive list of anthropological equipment that requires calibration: calipers (sliding, spreading, digital), osteometric board, mandibulometer, measuring tape (yes, the plastic tape used to measure long bone circumference requires calibration), MicroScribe digitizer or other three-dimensional data collection technology, thermometers used on processing equipment (i.e. incubator or steam kettle), and any microscope equipped with a micrometer or other length measuring device.

Equipment should be calibrated, if possible, by a qualified external calibration vendor who is accredited to ISO/IEC 17025. A laboratory calibration schedule should be established for each piece of equipment. A calibration check may be performed internally, in between external calibrations. For example, calipers can be internally checked by the Forensic Anthropologist using gage blocks every six months, while an external vendor is scheduled to visit the lab annually. If the equipment does not pass the internal calibration check, it should be taken out of service immediately and sent for external calibration. Documentation of calibration provides accountability and transparency; it establishes that the laboratory's equipment is functioning properly and that the results are reliable and accurate.

Other equipment for which calibration does not apply should still receive preventive maintenance or quality checks, as applicable. This includes non-measuring equipment, such as light microscopes, fume hoods, and radiography equipment (i.e. dental, medical, computerized tomography [CT]). Once again, documentation of regular, planned equipment maintenance demonstrates that the laboratory utilizes properly functioning, reliable (not to mention, safe) equipment.

While many anthropology laboratories now have QA measures, validation and verification of equipment and methods are the more challenging and less frequently discussed aspects of laboratory QA. "Although these terms may be used interchangeably, or with different meanings in other disciplines," as Pierce et al. (2016) explain, "they serve distinct purposes for assessing the validity of a method used by a forensic examiner." Validation assesses either a method or piece of equipment to determine whether its efficacy and reliability meet the requirements specified for its use in the laboratory (ISO/IEC 17025 2005). Verification assesses whether a method or procedure can be followed or applied adequately within the laboratory once validated (ISO 9000 2015). Verification, also referred to as internal validation, is conducted to demonstrate that a laboratory is precisely and reliably performing a method as detailed in the published literature or as implemented in another laboratory (Pierce et al. 2016).

As an example, the authors undertook validation and verification of two pieces of equipment at the HCIFS: the MicroScribe digitizer (and its associated software: 3Skull and Advantage Data Architect) and the Fordisc 3.1 software program. Although Forensic Anthropologists have used these items for years, and they are well-accepted data collection/analytical tools within the scholarly community, a formal validation from within the anthropology community could not be found. As an accredited laboratory, the Forensic Anthropologists had to demonstrate that the digitizer (Figure 5.1) and Fordisc software were functioning as intended, prior to implementation in forensic casework.

The internal validation of the MicroScribe digitizer involved multiple steps: (i) all anthropologists collected 42 osteometric landmarks on a pre-marked human cranium two separate times (i.e. repeatability or inter-observer data) to document that the digitizer was accurately capturing the three-dimensional data. (ii) These repeatability data were entered into a measurement uncertainty worksheet (see below) to calculate the amount of uncertainty associated with measurements derived from the digitizer. (iii) All anthropologists repeatedly (twice) collected 27 interlandmark distance measurements on the same pre-marked cranium using standard calipers to assess whether the digitizer was a comparable measurement tool. (iv) Technical error of measurement was calculated to evaluate whether the digitizer or calipers were more erroneous. (v) A risk assessment was conducted to determine the level of risk associated with the use of the digitizer. The acceptance criteria for this internal validation were as follows: (i) the digitizer transferred the craniometric and coordinate data into the 3Skull software program, and then

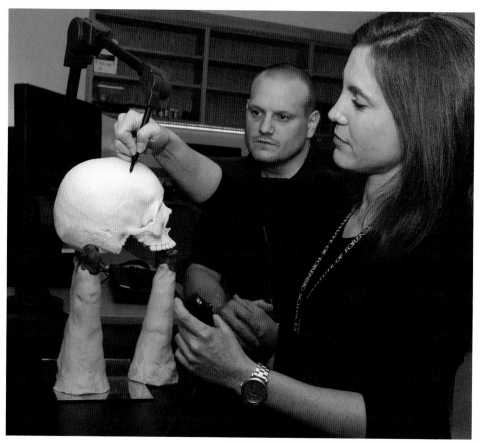

**Figure 5.1** Dr. Fleischman and Dr. Crowder testing theMicroScribe digitizer prior to conducting the internal validation study (Photograph by Andre Santos, HCIFS).

these data were transferred and opened in the Advantage Data Architect software without any errors; and (ii) the difference between the caliper and digitizer measurement value did not exceed ±2 mm. Since there is little data comparing caliper and digitizer measurements, the ±2 mm was chosen arbitrarily as an initial value for future guidance. If these criteria are met, the MicroScribe digitizer and the two associated software programs are functioning as prescribed and are valid.

The verification of the Fordisc 3.1 software required fewer steps: (i) eight craniometric and four postcraniometric datasets from individuals of known sex, ancestry, and stature were acquired from the donated human remains at the Forensic Anthropology Center at Texas State University. (ii) These data were input into the Fordisc software at the HCIFS and run with few, if any, transformations. (iii) The Fordisc results were compared with those that had been generated by the Fordisc software at Texas State. The acceptance criterion for this verification was as follows: in general, without running transformations or making complex analytical decisions, the ancestry, sex, and stature classifications produced with the Fordisc software at the HCIFS were reasonably similar to those produced by the Fordisc software at Texas State. Therefore, if two different laboratories, running two different copies of the Fordisc software, and analyzing the same data, generate similar ancestry, sex, and stature results, the software is working as intended and is valid.

Thus, in-house validation and verifications of analytical equipment, software, and methods are critical to demonstrate the level of surety associated with analyses. These aspects of QA are uncommon in anthropology, but we argue that they can and should be implemented in all Forensic Anthropology laboratories. Undergoing the process of validation and/or verification assists a laboratory in identifying any limitations of its equipment or software, as well as appropriate instructions to include in the SOP.

For some validation studies, specifically those that include measuring equipment, a laboratory can incorporate an assessment of measurement uncertainty. As indicated in laboratory accreditation programs, calculating and documenting the uncertainty of measurement for measuring processes is a standard component of measurement traceability that should be evaluated for critical measurements. Critical measurements are those that have a direct or significant effect on the accuracy or validity of a result or conclusion. Currently, there is not a clear manner for incorporating uncertainty of measurement values into multivariate analyses (i.e. cranial and postcranial measurements are entered into regression equations to generate ancestry, sex, or stature results); because the measurements do not produce results or conclusions without manipulation or analysis, it is debatable whether or not the standard Forensic Anthropological metrics are critical. Despite the issue of critical measurements, calculating uncertainty of measurement is an infrequently addressed aspect of QA in Forensic Anthropology laboratories, primarily because only three laboratories in the country are currently accredited. Estimating and documenting uncertainty of measurement demonstrates that the laboratory is cognizant of the variability in results derived from its measuring equipment and processes, and accounts for this variability when drawing analytical conclusions and writing medico-legal reports.

Uncertainty of measurement, however, is not synonymous with absolute error. Uncertainty relates to the dispersion of a measured value, often expressed in the form of a standard deviation or another expression of statistical distribution (Joint Committee for Guides in Metrology 2008b). As such, there is not one measured value "but an infinite number of values dispersed about the result that are consistent with all of the observations and data and one's knowledge of the physical world, and that with varying degrees of credibility can be attributed to the [object being measured]" (Joint Committee for Guides in Metrology 2008a). Conversely, error has numerous colloquial and scientific meanings. Error, as Christensen et al. (2014) explain, can be defined as: having false or incorrect information; a mistake or deviation in behavior; an assertion or act that unintentionally deviates from the truth; or, statistically and mathematically, the difference between a derived value and a true or theoretically correct value. For the purposes of QA in the laboratory setting, particularly when validating or verifying equipment or methods, assessing uncertainty is often more feasible than evaluating true error.

As such, the authors wanted to assess the magnitudes of measurement uncertainty for each piece of equipment used to measure human remains at their workplace, which includes sliding and spreading calipers, a measuring tape, the osteometric board, mandibulometer, and the MicroScribe digitizer. Adequately documenting uncertainty of measurement requires collecting various data, including reproducibility and repeatability (i.e. intra- and inter-observer error), equipment characteristics (i.e. values provided by the external vendor who calibrates the measuring equipment), and environmental factors (temperature, altitude, humidity, vibration, etc.). To collect the reproducibility and repeatability data, the Forensic Anthropologists collected multiple standardized measurements using each of the aforementioned measurement tools, similar to the MicroScribe validation procedure described above. These data, as well as the equipment characteristics and environmental factors, were entered into a spreadsheet that uses the root sum squares method to calculate the combined uncertainty of measurement of each measuring process. The spreadsheet also depicted which components of the measuring process were producing the most uncertainty. Not surprisingly, reproducibility and repeatability – the unintentional human errors — always had the most influence on measurement uncertainty.

But why, as forensic practitioners, and particularly as anthropologists, do we need to establish uncertainty of measurement (and error, in some cases)? As scientists who are regularly called to give expert testimony within the judicial system, Forensic Anthropologists should be able to demonstrate that they are aware of these scientific principles and that they can account for them in their results and reports. This awareness demonstrates to judges, lawyers, the jury, and other judicial entities, that anthropologists are intricately familiar with the state of forensic science and are pursuing higher standards. Perhaps more importantly, if questioned on the stand, Forensic Anthropologists can confidently state that they have estimated and documented their error or uncertainty – even if anthropological measurements are not deemed critical.

## 5.7   Implications of QA in the courtroom

### 5.7.1   Legal rulings affecting anthropology

The various legal rulings guiding the admissibility of scientific evidence and expert testimony – *Frye v. United States* (1923) and the 1975 Federal Rules of Evidence 702 (amended in the year 2000 in response to the Supreme Court's opinion in the *Daubert v. Merrell Dow Pharmaceuticals, Inc.* (1993) case) – must be considered when conducting Forensic Anthropological analyses and writing case reports. "Considering how law and science continue to converge," as Christensen and Crowder (2009) argue, "the science of anthropology … must be conceived under the rubric of evidentiary examination and methods need to be based on a sound scientific foundation with justifiable protocols." Similarly, the National Academy of Sciences' report (National Research Council 2009) states that an important question underlying legal admission and reliance upon forensic evidence is "the extent to which a particular forensic discipline is founded on a reliable scientific methodology that gives it the capacity to accurately analyze evidence and report findings." Thus, Forensic Anthropologists must strive to use methods, theories, and equipment/software that have been tested, that have known or potential error/uncertainty rates, that have standards of operation, that have been subjected to peer review and publication, and that are generally accepted within the scientific community (*Daubert v. Merrell Dow Pharmaceuticals, Inc.* 1993; Christensen and Crowder 2009).

As an expert witness, each Forensic Anthropologist must be able to convey that they are a qualified professional, but also that they are accurately using anthropological methods, theories, and equipment. A QA program "will help ensure the high quality of anthropological research, assist with establishing method transparency, and provide a secure foundation for Forensic Anthropologists in the courtroom" (Christensen and Crowder 2009). Returning to the example of uncertainty of measurement, even if the values generated by anthropological equipment are not deemed critical measurements, the HCIFS Forensic Anthropologists now have uncertainty of measurement calculations as part of their QA records and can provide them if requested by a court or other legal entity.

At both the laboratory and judicial levels, the implications of having a QA program for Forensic Anthropology are profound. Quality assurance neatly packages standards and oversight of personnel, training, equipment, and the procedures derived from methods/theories. This oversight and documentation limits errors in the laboratory, establishes the surety of the final conclusions and case reports, and ultimately provides transparency when Forensic Anthropologists are explaining their procedures and findings in a court of law.

## 5.8  Accreditation

While a QA program has internal implications for the Forensic Anthropologists, accreditation adds external merit to the program. Accreditation standards exist to set minimum requirements for those practicing in the same field and ultimately leads to a sense of uniformity between different agencies. Accreditation is for a service, not a person. Laboratory accreditation embodies not just the practitioners themselves, but also the infrastructure within which they work, including the QM system. Therefore, offices with one anthropologist are not precluded from obtaining accreditation, but the accreditation would not be solely for that person.

The major accrediting bodies for forensic disciplines use international standards – standards issued by the International Organization for Standardization (ISO) – as the backbone of their programs. ISO/IEC 17025 is the standard for laboratory testing and calibration. ISO/IEC 17020 is the standard for forensic inspection. Neither standard is superior to the other, as both foster a program for managing operations and serving customer needs. Those seeking accreditation should review both and determine which standard best suits their operation.

While an agency may not have the funds to obtain accreditation, it can still have an internal QA program that complies with accreditation requirements. Here is where having a separate QA group is helpful – QA personnel independent of the anthropology laboratory can objectively assess and monitor their compliance. For instance, one should not audit his/her own work. Separate QA personnel are in a better position to conduct an internal audit of the laboratory to provide feedback on the level of compliance and identify areas for improvement.

On the other hand, participating in the accreditation process is a true investment in quality and the future of the service. Allowing external auditors to assess your laboratory generates honest and objective feedback about the state of management and operations. Even if accreditation is not granted, the feedback is there to indicate areas requiring improvement. A laboratory can always work on improvements and reapply for accreditation at a later time.

Once accreditation is granted, the laboratory receives a certificate from the accreditation body that confirms compliance to its program standards. This would be an additional element of QA to discuss in court. Having a stamp of approval from an external body bolsters your agency's credibility and gives weight to your claim that you have an adequate QA program.

## 5.9  Conclusions

Achieving transparency in the forensic sciences encompasses many aspects of training and practice, managed and maintained through a robust QA program.

Quality assurance provides not only legal accountability, but makes sure forensic scientists are accountable to their office/university, their colleagues, and the
public, whom they serve. The QA program is designed to enable the division,
laboratory, and practitioner to function effectively and provide quality analyses
considering scientific, legal, and local community objectives. Disciplines, including Forensic Anthropology, can no longer operate outside of QA principles under
the guise of being a "soft" science. In the past, certain forensic disciplines received
a hall pass regarding QA; however, in light of court cases and congressional
pressure, we must break with the past and pursue a more standardized (i.e.
quality-oriented) future (see Chapter 2).

One tangible goal of a QA program is accreditation, and it is through accreditation that QA finds its "teeth" in the courtroom. An analyst may be the best in the
field and work at the largest laboratory; yet if they cannot demonstrate certified
competency and their laboratory holds no accreditations, there is less guarantee
of product quality. Considering that judges, with limited scientific background,
are the gatekeepers of scientific testimony, and jurors are laypeople who may
or may not understand the level of scrutiny associated with the scientific process, the ability to produce a stamp of approval is a concept that everyone can
appreciate.

If the Forensic Anthropology community works together, we can achieve
higher standards in our laboratories, universities, and offices, and embrace QA.
Although these concepts may seem daunting, sharing SOPs, developing com-
petency/proficiency tests for distribution, designing more uniform training programs, and encouraging accreditation are all steps we can take to improve our
science and support transparency in our laboratories and the courtroom.

# References

Christensen, A.M. and Crowder, C.M. (2009). Evidentiary standards for Forensic Anthro-
pology. *Journal of Forensic Sciences* 54 (6): 1211–1216.
Christensen, A.M., Crowder, C.M., Ousley, S.D., and Houck, M.M. (2014). Error and its
meaning in forensic science. *Journal of Forensic Sciences* 59 (1): 123–126.
*Daubert v. Merrell Dow Pharmaceuticals, Inc.*, 509 U.S. 579 (1993).
Deming, W.E. (1950). *Elementary Prinicples of the Statistical Control of Quality*. Union of
Japanese Scientists and Engineers (JUSE).
*Frye v. United States.* 293 F. 1013 (D.C. Cir. 1923).
ISO 9000. (2015). *Quality management systems—fundamentals and vocabulary* (5e). Geneva:
International Organization for Standardization.
ISO/IEC 17000. (2004). *Conformity assessment – Vocabulary and general principles, 3.2.*
Geneva: International Organization for Standardization/International Electrotechnical
Commission.
ISO/IEC 17025. (2005). *General requirements for the competence of testing and calibration
laboratories* (2e). Geneva: International Organization for Standardization/International
Electrotechnical Commission.

Joint Committee for Guides in Metrology. (2008a). Evaluation of measurement data: Guide to the expression of uncertainty in measurement (GUM). https://www.iso .org/sites/JCGM/GUM/JCGM100/C045315e-html/C045315e.html?csnumber=50461 (accessed March 31, 2018).

Joint Committee for Guides in Metrology. (2008b). International vocabulary of metrology: Basic and general concepts and associated terms (VIM). https://www.iso.org/sites/ JCGM/VIM/JCGM_200e.html (accessed March 31, 2018).

National Research Council (2009). *Strengthening Forensic Science in the United States: A Path Forward*. Washington, DC: National Academies Press.

Pierce, M.L., Wiersema, J.M., and Crowder, C.M. (2016). Progress in the accreditation of anthropology laboratories. *Academic Forensic Pathology* 6 (3): 344–348.

Shewhart, W.A. (1939). *Statistical Method from the Viewpoint of Quality Control*. Washington, DC: Graduate School of the Department of Agriculture.

# CHAPTER 6

# Report writing and case documentation in forensic anthropology

Lauren Zephro[1] and Alison Galloway[2]

[1] Santa Cruz County Sheriff's Office, Santa Cruz, CA, USA
[2] University of California, Santa Cruz, Santa Cruz, CA, USA

The forensic anthropological case report documents how and why a case was examined, the work done on a case, the observations and interpretations of data obtained from the remains and the professional opinion of the expert, or experts, who prepare the report. When completed, the final report should be sufficient to allow another qualified Forensic Anthropologist to assess the quality and thoroughness of the work done and the basis for conclusions drawn.

The foundation for such a final report starts not with the writing of the report, but on the case documentation in the form of observations made and preserved using photographs, notes, and worksheets. The report also lies within a context for professional standards, either from professional organizations or accrediting bodies that oversee the laboratory.

This chapter is written from the working perspectives of a crime-laboratory-based Forensic Anthropologist and an academically based Forensic Anthropologist. The perspectives brought to this chapter are shaped by the related non-anthropology duties, experience in the courtroom and the composition of casework. Dr. Zephro's perspective is that of a Forensic Laboratory Director, in charge of anthropological and non-anthropological forensic disciplines. Her perspective on casework is informed by quality management principles and standards of practice that have emerged from other forensic disciplines. Dr. Galloway has spent the majority of her career as a university-based Forensic Anthropologist, working as a consultant for defense counsel and the prosecution, as well as instructing and mentoring students in Forensic Anthropology. Her role as a neutral player in evaluating evidence has been seasoned by her non-law-enforcement-based position and casework, which treats and accepts prosecution cases and defense cases with equal attention.

*Forensic Anthropology and the United States Judicial System*, First Edition.
Edited by Laura C. Fulginiti, Kristen Hartnett-McCann, and Alison Galloway.
© 2019 John Wiley & Sons Ltd. Published 2019 by John Wiley & Sons Ltd.

We recognize that our positions represent only two of the many positions that Forensic Anthropologists may occupy. These roles, based on agency policy, procedure and expectations, may potentially change the requirements for documentation and reporting from a Forensic Anthropologist, and may require use of specific formats. While not all reporting structures can be covered in a single chapter, the principles of clarity, transparency, and accuracy should pervade all reports.

In this chapter, we begin with the basics of why case reports are produced and what purpose they serve to their various audiences, now and in the future. In addition, we lay out the package of documents that should be expected with Forensic Anthropology case reports including the written opinion of the expert and the supporting documentation.

## 6.1   The audience(s)

It is important to understand that the Forensic Anthropology case report has an extensive reach and must, therefore, be suitable for several different audiences. First, the report provides a format for the anthropologist to lay out their approach to a case, their observations and conclusions, and what supporting documentation should be expected if discovery of the case file is requested. The report should also serve as a checklist to ensure that the anthropologist has thought through the conclusions and has also addressed all the basic areas. Using the report as a form of a checklist can also act as a guide to make sure that no relevant information is missed.

Secondly, investigators working a case need the information in order to begin the search for the identity of the decedent and to distinguish what type of investigatory resources are needed and at what speed they need to be deployed. For example, an active homicide investigation requires significant resources to be deployed immediately, whereas a case where the bones are determined to be historic, will not require a full-blown criminal investigation. The information the audience will need should be quickly and clearly stated.

Thirdly, if this is indeed a criminal case for which there will be prosecution of an alleged perpetrator, then the report is included in the information given to the district attorney when the case is filed. If for no other reason, the district attorney will need this information to lay the groundwork for a case – that a homicide has actually been committed and the investigation addressed all possible avenues, regardless of who is accused. In these situations, the district attorney needs to understand the limitations of the information. For example, what is the expected interval for the estimated time since death or what do we mean by "perimortem"? Significantly, most audiences of forensic case reports do not have a background in

Forensic Anthropology, so automatically, our report has a teaching component. As scientists, we have a duty to clarify our terms and meanings, so what we think we say in a report is interpreted within the accepted limits of our discipline.

Fourthly, if a case is going to prosecution, the report is handed to the defense team of attorneys and investigators to review. If the defense team needs to question the findings or evaluate whether the overall investigatory work was comprehensive, unbiased, and appropriate, then the report will go to another anthropologist. Because ours is a small community, most practicing Forensic Anthropologists know each other's work and also know each other. Many share professors or students. This familiarity means that a colleague, mentor, or student is being asked to dissect our report. Although having a colleague critically evaluate a report and/or case file may be difficult, work done in the forensic realm is not about the expert but rather about the victims and suspects, families and communities, and the legal community representing the invested parties. These parties have no other way to evaluate the quality of work than to seek their own expert to assess the examination of remains and resulting conclusions.

Finally, the report stands as a court document that will likely be entered into evidence. The work of the anthropologist is often critical in determining that a crime was committed and when it probably occurred. Additionally, the report can form the basis for arguments about findings in other cases, most notably that of the pathologist.

## 6.2   The report begins with documentation of workflow

No report can rectify errors made during the analysis so understanding and following standard laboratory procedures is important. Standard operating procedures (SOPs) should be available in every laboratory. Rather than a rigid guideline, these should document the practices of the laboratory and allow for the flexibility needed when a given case does not fit within the standard framework. SOPs provide documentation for what you should do, how you should approach things, how to record the results and the basic interpretations. They do not hamper what can be done but do provide baselines. Procedures should also be upgraded as the anthropologist modifies practice to meet new techniques, technology, or professional standards.

The workflow in the laboratory begins with a request for services, whether for recovery of material from a crime scene or for material brought to the anthropology laboratory. Figure 6.1 charts a sample workflow of a Forensic Anthropology case and the primary types of documentation that will be collected at each stage, initiated as a request to investigate a crime scene. Figure 6.2 represents the same requirements that would accompany a request for services

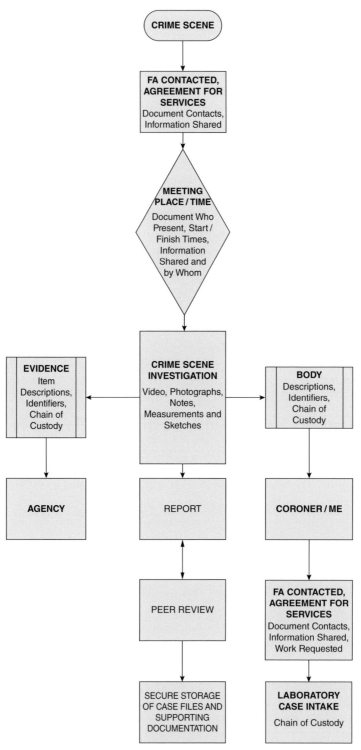

**Figure 6.1** Workflow for scene recovery and documentation.

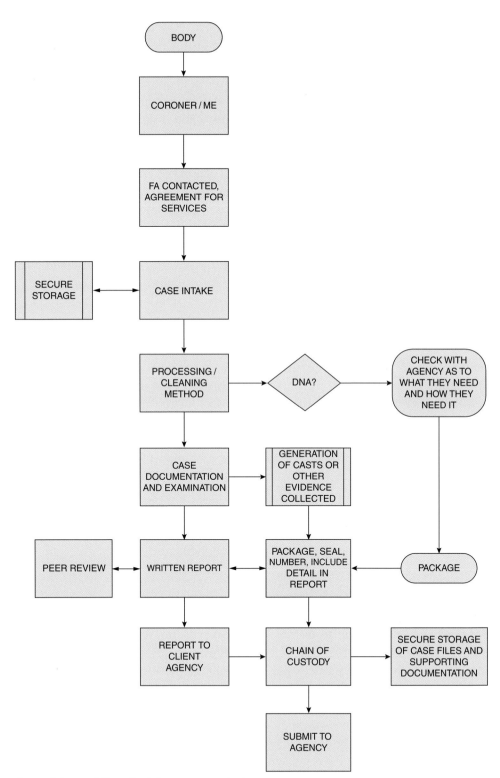

**Figure 6.2** Workflow for laboratory analysis.

that involve the laboratory analysis of remains. Prior to the submission of a case however, it is ideal that there is a pre-existing relationship between the Forensic Anthropologist and client agency, that includes a review of credentials, expectations, services provided, how to contact in an emergency, etc., along with a fee schedule for work performed. Obviously, depending on where the anthropologist works and agency or institutional requirements, the above relationship and expectations may differ.

When a case is accepted, it needs to be accompanied with agency documentation, including the case number and agency contact information, and there should be clear expectations as to the types of services needed. Has the identification of the individual been established positively or tentatively? Is the request limited to an assessment of traumatic defects? If there is an expectation for postmortem interval assessment, have the photographs and other necessary information (location, conditions, and date/time found) been provided? The anthropologist must become the manager of information (see below).

## 6.3   Chain of custody

The transfer of remains to the anthropologist must be accompanied by a chain of custody form. At a minimum, this form includes the agency and case number, the items being transferred and the reason for the transfer, the name and signature of the person who is providing the material and same for the person who is receiving the material, along with the date and time of the transfer. This chain supports the beginning sections of the case report by documenting what and when the material arrived for anthropological examination. It should also include the storage location(s) with date/time and reason for transfer within the laboratory, if needed. All those with direct handling of the remains should be identified in the chain or case notes. All those with access to the case while in the anthropologist's custody are subject to subpoena.

## 6.4   Managing the information flow

We need the information to do our jobs, however, too much information may inadvertently bias our observations and conclusions. The potential pitfall of bias requires us to be active participants in managing when and what information comes to us.

Bias, which has recently emerged a premier topic of research and discussion in forensic science, is the trickiest of all phenomena because it is not a conscious phenomenon. We do not consciously know when we are selectively assessing material based on preconceived notions. Bias requires us to take a proactive stance in documenting what we knew, when we knew it, and from whom did the information come. Our cases may benefit from knowing as little as possible about the presumed circumstances of death and suspected identity. To have the opportunity, if only for the first few minutes at a crime scene or looking at a bone without any preconceived ideas, can make a huge difference in our ability to be better examiners. Managing and limiting the flow of external information can take the form of many smaller actions. For example, a good policy requires a first walk-through of a scene to be conducted without a synopsis of what law enforcement thinks happened, or to whom they think the remains might belong.

Recent research has offered a striking glimpse of the potential strength of contextually biasing information on forensic anthropological examinations (Nakhaeizadeh et al. 2014, 2018). Law enforcement often provides information to the anthropologist including who the decedent might be or what they think might have happened, despite measures taken to limit exposure to additional context. For example, an investigator may start the request with "we think it is a 24-year-old woman that has been missing for two years." This comment already implants sufficient information that it may mask some details or steer the anthropologist toward certain conclusions – not through intent but through cognitive bias. Unfortunately, it is possible that the evidence will be interpreted to conform to this scenario, thereby ignoring information that does not fit the desired outcome. In this circumstance, the anthropologist is essentially trying to work backwards from a conclusion instead of having their conclusions dictated solely by their observations, and this may lead them inadvertently to erroneous conclusions or mistakes. Therefore, any such information that is received should be noted in the lab bench notes or communication log. A communication log is a simple document, recording when conversations or consultations occurred, and what information was shared, by whom and when. It can be a standard form in the case file. Sharing expectations for information transmission can also be discussed with the clients prior to case submissions, so that expectations are set and minimal explanations are needed when working on an actual case.

There are specific pieces of information that are important, particularly if the request for analysis includes an estimation of the postmortem interval. Along with the remains, the anthropologist will need information on the context of the recovery. Basic information should include:
- Date and time of discovery/recovery.
- Exact location of recovery such as a street address, milepost, or GPS coordinates.
- Circumstances of the remains (buried, surface scatter, under brush, in a structure, in a box, etc.).

- Photographs showing the body at the time of recovery and, if the body is covered, photographs from autopsy showing sufficient body surface to assess decomposition.

## 6.5    Processing the remains and storage considerations

SOPs should prescribe the processing and storage of the remains and the case report should provide the key points of the processing of the material in order to get it ready for analysis. The details, however, are usually documented in the SOPs. These policies determine whether material is macerated, placed in a dermestid beetle colony and/or placed in hot water baths with either degreasers or detergents. The SOPs should also provide guidelines for why different processes may be used for different segments of the remains, depending on the time allowed for preparation. In some case, some portions of the remains will be held without processing in order to preserve material for DNA analysis, which should be noted in the case record.

The actual analysis of the remains should also follow a standard format, with some flexibility depending on the material available. How the body is examined should be documented including use of magnification, alternate light sources, radiographic/CT scans, casting, or other imaging techniques. Photographs of bones should be made showing multiple views, especially when there are indications of anomalous conditions, pathological conditions, and traumatic defects. Additionally, casts or other images produced may result in laboratory created evidence, which requires documentation and chain of custody, as these materials may be submitted to the law enforcement agency for retention.

## 6.6    Contemporaneous bench notes and standard forms

Once the processing, examination, and analysis is complete, what documents should the completed case file contain? Documents form the foundation upon which the case report is based and serves to refresh memories when this case comes to trial, often years after the report was written. In the modern forensic laboratory, it is inappropriate for observations or conclusions to be documented in a report but not in bench notes recorded contemporaneously to the examination. Bench notes do not support the report, the report supports the bench notes. This represents a significant departure from how much forensic anthropological casework was conducted and how documentation was produced in the recent past.

For the anthropologist working in the academic setting or as an independent consultant, most records will be handwritten. For those working in larger laboratory settings, laboratory information management systems (LIMSs) are used by many crime laboratories, Coroner and Medical Examiner's offices. This software manages the information flow and collection from the lab request, into lab, assignment of material to different people, support forms and note forms, reports and much more.

The security of these notes must also be considered. For paper records, locked file cabinets with limited and known access should be used. For digital records, there are in-house and Cloud-based storage solutions that meets government security requirements. For the academic anthropologist, university IT departments can often provide information about secured Cloud-based storage, often available through the university which, itself, has huge needs for secured storage of records.

Information in the file will typically include the following items:
- Copies of the initial request, such as phone notes or emails.
- Chain of custody transfer form (or photographs of the form if copying facilities are not available).
- Correspondence with agency requesting service.
- Scene sketches, measurements, and charts if scene recovery included.
- Scene personnel log.
- Field notes from scene recovery.
- Skeletal inventory chart or list.
- Checklists/observations on sex, age, ancestry, stature, and measurements.
- Observations on anomalies, pathologies, and trauma or other damage to the skeleton.
- Activity log documenting processing.
- Photography log or contact sheet.

Inevitably, there will be errors made in the notes. At a minimum, these should be indicated by a single line strikeout and initialed or initialed and dated, depending on laboratory policy. While tempting, items cannot be simply discarded and new items substituted.

One of the biggest concerns about the notes and forms is what is discoverable and the answer is simple, everything, aside from a narrow band of material that would fall under attorney work product, is discoverable. This work product only refers to the interactions between the lawyer and the expert in preparation for the case – such as potential questions – and can, therefore, be excluded. Peer review feedback may or may not be included in the final case file per laboratory policy (as long as the work done conforms to laboratory standards), once changes have been made or incorporated into the final report.

Lastly, all the hard copy supporting documentation in the case file should be given page numbers out of a total number of pages, date, case number, and initials. Any digital documentation or other materials generated must also be documented in the case file. By taking this approach, future consumers of the work will know if there is any case file material missing when provided materials to review.

## 6.7    Casting, radiography, and other methods of documentation

Not all evidence generated in the context of a case analysis will be in the form of documents and charts. Radiographs, scans, three-dimensional images, and casts are also parts of the record. For example, there may be silicone casts made of tool marks on bone in order to present and preserve evidence of sharp force trauma that would be lost if the body is repatriated to the family. It is important to note that making a cast of a bone creates evidence. This new, laboratory-created evidence requires a chain of custody and documentation on how and why it came to be. The laboratory-created evidence, unless it is specifically required to remain in the custody of the anthropologist, should be submitted to the client agency upon return of the remains.

## 6.8    The report

All the analysis and documentation and photography that is conducted in the analysis is designed to produce a solid, supportable case report. This document records how and why the case was presented for analysis, what information was provided along with the case, the fundamentals of the case in terms of the bio-logical profile, the analysis of the trauma and the assessment of the postmortem interval. It states the opinions and conclusions reached as a result of the analysis and should be readable by the various members of the audience that receive it.

Because of the level of scrutiny, every case report should reflect the professionalism that has been brought to the case in general. The level of care given to the report is often an indication of the level of care given to the analysis. Ethical standards require that statements not only be accurate within the profession but also not be misleading to the lay reader.

### 6.8.1    Format of the case report

The case report is a formal document but there is no consistent format to which one should adhere. Indeed, these are often documents that evolve over time as new expectations are incorporated or where feedback leads to improvements. For the Forensic Anthropologist working for a federal, state, or local agency, there may be a standard format used by the agency. As long as the information that needs to be imparted can be accommodated into that template, then there should be no problem using a standard format.

Many anthropologists, however, work out of educational institutions or as separate consultants. In those cases, the development of a case report format is more idiosyncratic. Many use a "report" or "letter" format, some with a title page or cover. If the letter format is used, formal stationery is customary, particularly if the work is done as part of the service component of their university or college employment.

The report should include the following basics: your name, the agency requesting service, the agency case number, the anthropologist's case number if using a separate numbering system, and the date of the report. Some anthropologists also include a standard presentation of their qualifications so that the various members of the reading audience become familiar with the merits of the presentation. If included, this section should summarize the main points as a full curriculum vitae will be required if the matter proceeds further.

### 6.8.2 Background

Providing a description of how the anthropologist became involved, how and what information they learned and a basic understanding of the type of remains usually forms the first section. If the anthropologist was involved at the scene, then the process of recovery should be documented. This description would include when and where the recovery occurred, the personnel involved (including the names and agencies of those personnel met at the scene), what processes were involved in the search such as spiral search, grid search on hands and knees, or cadaver dogs. How were the bones exposed and what screening processes were used? What items of evidence were associated? What was the soil condition, moisture, and vegetation in the area? Were there insects present or vestiges of their earlier activity? Was there evidence of scavenging by animals or movement of the body by other means? Was the body scattered or articulated, what type of covering, if any, was present, and where were the bones in relation to other items of evidence?

If the anthropologist was responsible for mapping the overall scene, then sketches and measurements should be included. In many cases, agencies will work in tandem with the anthropologist to handle the overall sketch. Excavation depictions and profiles produced by the anthropologist during the recovery should be included. Sometimes these figures can be included in the body of the report but often, due to the extensive nature of the material, they fit better as an appendix. If adding an appendix, figures should be noted in the report so that readers know to refer to an appendix to see the depiction.

When the body arrives at the laboratory, either following the anthropologist-involved scene recovery or directly from the agency, the report should note the condition of the material transferred to the custody of the laboratory. This information should reflect the transfer of custody form so, if the remains come in a large body bag, a paper bag containing the skull and a plastic tub labeled as containing the throat, the report should so state and the transfer form should have three items. Since all such containers need to be noted and records reflect the contents, the documentation of such material can be lengthy. Often, when opening one bag, there are many more bags, envelopes, or vials inside, each with a number. There may also be additional inclusions such as copies of reports or radiographs. Again, appendices are a great way to provide these, often extensive, lists.

Business cards from the personnel involved are handy when it comes to preparing the report. While the exchange of business cards seems to be a courtesy when accepting information, it is a chance to get the correct spelling of the person's name and their official title and affiliation. This exchange allows the report to reflect the number and identity of others involved in the scene or delivery.

Much of the information about the case recovery is included in documentation that comes from the contracting agency in the form of photographs, investigator reports, and autopsy reports. Such information is useful in preparation of the case and report but, as the anthropologist does not have first-hand knowledge of this information, the term "reportedly" tends to be used extensively when introducing and integrating the outside information into the anthropology report. For example, the report would state that the remains are "reportedly identified by DNA analysis."

What information the anthropologist received prior to conducting the examination should be included in the report background section. This information speaks to the possibility of cognitive bias (see Section 6.4) – how foreknowledge of information may have influenced the final determinations. This information should be presented and should reflect the communications or activity log information.

### 6.8.3  Condition of the remains

Once the background information is completed, the report should cover the overall condition of the body. Obviously, the remains are likely to have changed between the time of discovery and arrival at the laboratory for anthropological analysis but this information does allow the reader to understand what those changes were and what the anthropologist saw at the initiation of the analysis. Was the body skeletonized, mummified, fully fleshed, etc.? Was there any information on more than one individual involved? A skeletal inventory should be presented, either as a table of presence and absence or a chart of the skeleton showing the portions present and absent. If more than a single individual is present, then the distinction between individuals and which bones cannot be assigned with confidence must also be noted. If the bones submitted are few in number, then the bones can simply be listed. This is often the case when a single cranium or skull is examined.

One advantage of using a chart for the skeletal inventory is that it can also be used to mark trauma or postmortem damage. This overview is useful for court presentation as the jury can understand the extent of damage and on what the anthropologist had to base their opinions. Typically, the views are an anterior and posterior skeleton, or anterior/posterior/right and left sides of the skeleton.

### 6.8.4  Biological profile

As we move into the results of the analysis, it is appropriate to shift the writing to the present tense. This shift seems awkward at first but there is a legal reason for doing so. If the past tense is used, an opposing attorney may suggest that the results were one way when examination occurred but may change when re-examined. Use of the present tense supposes that the determinations are still in force as in "this body is that of a male" as opposed to "was that of a male." If the use of the past tense is preferred, it must be used consistently and check with the client agency for preference.

If the biological profile is needed, the determination of sex, age, ancestry, and stature should be noted. For each, a brief description of why this determination was made should be included in the report. This information allows the expert retained by the opposing attorneys to assess the validity of the interpretation. Lack of such information stalls the assessment of the report until it can be delivered. Typically, bench notes are used to support these interpretations in that the findings should be included in notes.

The thoroughness of the biological profile depends on whether the remains have already been identified and the level of that identification (positive vs. circumstantial). If the person has already been identified and that information has been released to the anthropologist, the report should address the consistency between the observations and the identity. For example, one could say that the remains are those of a young adult female of mixed ancestry with an estimated height of 5'1"–5'5", consistent with the reported identity of the body as (give the name). If there are inconsistencies, these should also be noted.

When the body is unidentified, then the report should list as much suitable information for assisting with identity as possible. Sex, age, ancestry, and stature should be listed with the appropriate range highlighted. Often people present a summary of the pertinent facts as a table early in the report. However, the justification behind these determinations should be present in the report. Older styles of reports tended to be very brief, such as simply stating that the sex is male, but newer styles, along with expectations for peer review, require that supporting information be present. Why was the sex determination made as male? What skeletal features were noted consistent with this, and were any inconsistent? What methods were used? Was metric analysis undertaken? For age and stature, the confidence interval is used rather than the mean. Mean values tend to focus attention on a single number and may cause agencies to discount a close possible match.

For anomalies that appear on the remains, those that would appear radiographically, alter body function, or would have been noticeable in life, should be noted in the report. Bodies have many anomalous conditions that are of interest to anthropologists because there are possible genetic tendencies that allow us to look at possible kinship in archeological collections. However, in the forensic setting, these conditions may not be helpful to the agencies and should not be detailed.

Similarly, pathological conditions that should have led to medical treatment, produced noticeable pain to the victim, or that could have contributed to their demise, should be described and possible etiologies listed. For example, significant arthritis in one joint or set of joints, disproportionate to that found elsewhere in the body, may be a condition noted in missing person's reports or be recognizable to family and friends.

Often, in the pathological conditions noted, there will be a number of dental problems. Normally a forensic odontologist should have been consulted by the agency but it is also useful for the anthropologist to include a dental chart. The dental chart serves a double function of recording which teeth are present at the time of examination and anthropological observations on teeth that may relate to habits, age, ancestry, sex, anomaly, or disease. These features may be outside the scope of a forensic odontology report. The timing of loss for teeth should be noted as to whether they were missing antemortem or postmortem. Chips and fractures on teeth may also be helpful for identification while those of recent origin may be due to trauma or postmortem damage.

Figures are very helpful in providing the full context of the anomalies and pathologies seen in the remains. These images may be less useful to the lay person but will assist another anthropologist in understanding the attention drawn to this condition.

### 6.8.5   Trauma analysis

The trauma section is often one of the two most critical portions of the report in the long term as it is used in those cases where the cause and manner of death needs to be determined by the coroner or medical examiner and where, if a homicide, there will be court proceedings. The primary focus will be on the perimortem defects. In some reports, anthropologists list all trauma in this section while others prefer to list antemortem with biological profile and postmortem with the postmortem interval.

The determination of antemortem, perimortem, and postmortem traumatic defects should include a clear description of what this terminology means in the anthropological sense. Too often, investigators and attorneys assume that "perimortem" in the anthropological sense refers to events that occurred within minutes of the victim's demise rather than, as is the case in skeletal analysis, from a week or two before death to possibly months after death.

Standardized text describing "antemortem," "perimortem," and "postmortem" is useful to include in the trauma section of all reports. One such example is given in the following paragraph:

> There are three periods of skeletal trauma. Antemortem trauma is defined as bone damage sustained prior to death, showing clearly recognizable signs of healing. Perimortem skeletal trauma is defined as bone damage that displays fracture characteristics consistent with fresh bone with no indications of healing. Skeletal perimortem trauma may include bone trauma that occurs up to about two weeks before death and after death until postmortem fracture characteristics or events can be discerned. Postmortem trauma is defined as bone damage that occurs after the bone has lost the characteristics of fresh bone.

This description allows discussion of the antemortem defects as those that show signs of healing rather than those occurring up until the time the person stopped breathing. Because this antemortem period can be up to a couple of weeks prior to the actual death during which time there may not be initiation of visible skeletal healing, it is essential that this foundation be laid in every report on trauma. Attorneys may not be cognizant of the distinctions anthropologists make as opposed to those made by the pathologist.

It is equally important to understand that postmortem defects can only be distinguished by a complex of characteristics that are often difficult to identify. Some defects are categorized due to the mechanism of production such as carnivore damage and others can be identified by features such as lack of staining or soil within the fracture margin. Others depend on dryness of the margin producing a frayed appearance, excessive cracking and more brittleness. However, it is difficult to actually classify accuracy on these determinations based on single features (Wieberg and Wescott 2008; Zephro 2012).

The other standard section that is helpful in a report is a basic set of terms that distinguish the various points where traumatic damage occurs. Often each defect can be interpreted as a separate blow when, in fact, several defects can be produced by a single imposition of force to the bone. Again, a standardized paragraph can help explain this designation. For example, the following text would be appropriate:

> The trauma documented in this report will be described in terms of defects, fractures and insults. A **defect** is an imperfection on the bone, a failure or absence of bones or bony features. A **fracture** is a specialized type of defect in which there is traumatic rupture of the integrity of the bone, and an **insult** is the causal event of one or more defects
>
> *(Galloway and Zephro 2005).*

Whatever the approach or set of terms used, it is important to be consistent in the description of trauma. If using some text like the above paragraph, then a number of defects seen should be noted first, then grouped together as an insult or impact point. The mechanisms for the production of each defect should be listed. For example, "Defect B is a greenstick fracture of the left 7th rib located at the midpoint of the shaft. Transverse fracturing occurs on the external surface, consistent with anteroposterior compression of the ribcage."

Once the defects are listed, then the possible number of insults needs to be determined. Using the above example, if the right ribs 7 through 9 all have similar fractures and these are all in about the same location, then one insult is possible, producing multiple fractures. Often these fractures will actually align when the ribs are placed back in anatomical position. Similar alignments are often seen in dismemberment cases where decapitation efforts produce defects to the neck and mandible. It is, therefore, important to think beyond the immediate segment of the body but the range of placements of limbs and other segments.

Images are often critical in communicating about traumatic defects. While the chart of the skeletal inventory can show the overall locations of defects on the skeleton, the actual defect should be shown in a separate figure. Sometimes, as with rib injuries, it is helpful to have the defects alongside a diagram of the rib cage. Again, there are differences of opinion as to whether these images should be added as an appendix or included in the report.

Trauma to the cranium or cranium and mandible are common findings in forensic cases. These defects are often critical in cases where homicide is suspected. In court, presentation with the actual skeletal material may occur but, in most cases, the communication with the jury rests on the photographs. A six-view composite photographic figure showing the front, back, both sides, superior and inferior views is useful and three-dimensional renderings are increasingly being included. Unfortunately, defects are often small or masked by decompositional fluids so close-up photos, linked to the overall and midrange photographs, may be crucial. Often a tracing of the six-view composite, with labels for the defects and areas of insult, is also extremely useful in explaining the injury patterns, including sequence, where fractures linked to one blow can be color coded and distinguished from other areas of damage.

Cause and manner of death fall outside the purview of the Forensic Anthropologist. The anthropological summary of the trauma should focus on the number of defects, the number of insults and the mechanism of production such as blunt force impact, sharp force impact or high velocity projectile impact. Direction of impact should be included. Linkage between injuries is important. For example, injuries on one side of the head may be due to direct blows while those on the other side may be due to compression of the head resting on a substrate at the time of the impacts on the opposite side. Injuries to the knee in a victim of a motor vehicle driver may be related to the shearing fracture at the femoral neck and posterior acetabulum from the entire leg being driven backwards. The summary of the trauma should lay out the possible relationship between injuries, given the anatomical constraints of the body.

### 6.8.6 Postmortem interval and the time since death

The final substantive section of the report focuses on the duration of the postmortem interval and what might have occurred to the body during that period. First, the discussion should state at what time the observations are made and the data upon which the determinations are calculated. In some cases, the observations are made on the remains as they arrived in the laboratory. This is common with mummified or skeletonized remains. However, since bodies often decay considerably between the time of recovery and arrival at the anthropologist's laboratory, the anthropologist often needs to rely on photographs taken during the recovery process if they did not participate in the recovery. This is particularly the case when the body has been recovered with sufficient soft tissue to allow an autopsy. In these cases, photographs taken at autopsy are often used to supplement scene recovery photos that may not reveal the needed body segments for assessment. In any of these cases, the report must clearly state what was used (including image numbers), how and from whom they were obtained, and what they reportedly show. Since we are usually relying on images we did not take ourselves, we cannot vouch for their accuracy directly so the term "reportedly" is often attached to descriptions of the photograph as in "the photograph reportedly shows the remains at the time they were pulled from the sand."

Discussion of the postmortem interval typically looks at the overall changes to the remains and the estimate based on the anthropologist's experience with the local environments. Like the other numerical estimates, a time interval (weeks, months, or years) is given of the most likely time that death occurred.

In many cases, this decomposition estimate is paralleled by a calculation based on accumulated degree days. Again, if the source of the total body score is the photographs obtained from the agency and reportedly taken at recovery, then that information should be noted. Then, the anthropologist should note where the weather data was obtained, usually a National Oceanic and Atmospheric Administration website. The relationship between the location of the weather station in relation to the site of recovery should be presented in both distance but also, if known, environment. Then the report states from what date the calculation is made and by whose formula the calculation was made. Because this is a complicated process, it is often good to lay out the steps in associated tables so that it can be followed by the various readers. The results are usually provided as dates within the confidence intervals, rather than the broader categories of the gross observations.

### 6.8.7   Report summary and disposition

The report concludes with a quick summary of the findings. This allows those who need a concise check to quickly locate that and provides a short quote of the case that can be used in future communications. In addition, this is the time to state what will be done with the evidence – the body, photographs, notes, digital records and all the other material accumulated in the course of the analysis. For example, the report may state:

> Photographs, notes and digital records will be archived at the XXXX Laboratory. Skeletal material is retained by XXXX Laboratory until arrangements for return to the Coroner's Office can be made.

## 6.9   Appendices

References included in the report, such as the formula used in the postmortem interval determination, can be added as an appendix to the report. This is usually not a lengthy list, remember the anthropologist is responsible for knowing inside and out all the data upon which he or she relies. This is also not a scholarly work so citing everything that has been published on a topic is not appropriate.

Other appendices, depending on preference, can include the photographs and figures, charts of the inventory and tables for measurements. Some include the Forensic Databank forms as part of their report. Worksheets are included by some but are not needed as they remain part of the case evidence and are discoverable if needed.

One appendix that is increasingly being included is a brief biography of the anthropologist. While the agency requesting service may well have a copy of the curriculum vitae, the biography allows other members of the audience to know the background of the report writer. Such documents are often required in international jurisdictions and will probably become necessary within the United States.

## 6.10   Final steps

All reports should be signed and each page should be initialed. Some agencies also require a witness to countersign the signature of the anthropologist to ensure that it is submitted by the person stated. If multiple people are involved and all signing the report, then it should not be submitted until all signatures are complete. Paper copies are often sent back with the remains or mailed separately but electronic communication is the norm for most agencies. Draft copies are usually sent electronically.

Once the report is completed to the satisfaction of all the people involved in it, it is ready for the first outside audience, peer review (see Chapter 8). Peer review is now an important part of case work and report writing. Exchange of reports between professionals allows for better clarity and for areas where there may be controversy to be identified early. Frequently, there are minor modifications that the reviewer will request such as "this wording sounds ambiguous" or "you seem to be missing a caption."

Most anthropologists have an exchange program set up with standardized comment pages on their response to a report. This form addresses what was reviewed, whether it meets the technical standards, whether there are issues of clarity or consistency that should be addressed and, finally, whether there are additional issues such as typographical errors. Because these are signed, the reviewer is also accepting a level of responsibility in the submission of the report in that they are putting behind the work their reputation that it is valid.

Preservation of the records is an important but often overlooked requirement of the profession. Fundamental to this concern is the question of to whom do the records belong. While they are the work product of the anthropologist, they ultimately belong to the agency responsible for the investigation of the death.

The question of ownership comes to a head as a Forensic Anthropologist moves toward retirement or transition to another institution. Unless there is someone who is assuming the forensic functions of the laboratory, then material should be transferred to the contracting agency along with bench notes, email, photographs, and any other associated material.

Reports generated for the defense can be more problematic but at least digital copies of all material should be provided to the attorney who headed the defense so that it is available should another appeal be mounted.

## 6.11  Conclusion

Production of a case report is not an isolated process. Instead, it is the product of a careful approach to analysis, meticulous record-keeping and a dedication to transparency and high ethical standards. It stands as a lasting communication between the anthropologist and a broad audience of readers, whose interests differ widely.

## References

Galloway, A. and Zephro, L. (2005). Skeletal trauma analysis of the lower extremity. In: *Forensic Medicine of the Lower Extremity: Human Identification and Trauma Analysis of the Thigh, Leg and Foot* (ed. J. Rich, D.E. Dean and R.H. Powers), 249–273. Totowa, NJ: Humana Press.

Nakhaeizadeh, S., Dror, I.E., and Morgan, R.M. (2014). Cognitive bias in Forensic Anthropology: visual assessment of skeletal remains is susceptible to confirmation bias. *Science and Justice* 54: 208–214.

Nakhaeizadeh, S., Morgan, R.M., Rando, C., and Dror, I.E. (2018). Cascading bias of initial exposure to information at the crime scene to the subsequent evaluation of skeletal remains. *Journal of Forensic Sciences* 63 (2): 403–411.

Wieberg, D.A. and Wescott, D.J. (2008). Estimating the timing of long bone fractures: correlation between the postmortem interval, bone moisture content, and blunt force trauma fracture characteristics. *Journal of Forensic Sciences* 53 (5): 1028–1034.

Zephro, L. (2012). Determining the timing and mechanism of bone fracture. PhD dissertation. University of California, Santa Cruz.

# CHAPTER 7

# Skull shots: forensic photography for anthropologists

Lauren Zephro[1] and Alison Galloway[2]

[1] Santa Cruz County Sheriff's Office, Santa Cruz, CA, USA
[2] University of California, Santa Cruz, Santa Cruz, CA, USA

Photography in a forensic context provides a visual representation of evidence, from start to finish, documenting context, condition, process, and examination. Photographs illustrate the general condition and alterations of a scene or evidence and can be used in examination and comparison later in time. The photographs taken during the recovery process and the analytical processes usually are the ones that will be used in courtroom presentations. Photographs also form the primary means by which experts for opposing counsel will evaluate the findings in the forensic report. They are the window into the anthropological processes for the jury and should allow the jury to draw the same conclusions from what they see, together with the verbal testimony that the expert made (see Chapters 9 and 10). With the advent of new technology such as DNA comparisons, cold case investigations are becoming commonplace, revisiting cases 20 or 30 years after the initial investigation. Photographs not considered important at the time of the investigation may present relevant information during a review that may occur days, weeks, or even years later. Therefore, diligence in how these images are produced is essential.

Photography and videography are nondestructive but, as the visual record of proceedings, should be approached with planning and forethought. Digital imaging facilitates comprehensive coverage but quality and context are not automatic. With digital photography and videography, however, we have the added benefit of having immediate access to verify that what we meant to capture is what the camera recorded.

This chapter presents the basic equipment needed for production of courtroom quality images, how to frame and provide context in the images, and how to overcome problems of working on skeletal material. Basic principles of crime scene

*Forensic Anthropology and the United States Judicial System*, First Edition.
Edited by Laura C. Fulginiti, Kristen Hartnett-McCann, and Alison Galloway.
© 2019 John Wiley & Sons Ltd. Published 2019 by John Wiley & Sons Ltd.

**Table 7.1** Recommended photography equipment for scene response kit.

DSLR camera with interchangeable lenses, full frame or cropped sensor. High resolution
  preferred
Multipurpose lens (ex. 28–70 mm or 18–140 mm)
Macro lens for close-up images
Telephoto and wide-angle lens (optional but recommended)
Detachable flash with sync cord or wireless connectivity
Camera remote
Tripod
Scales, including L-scales
Memory cards
Additional charged batteries/battery charger

and laboratory photography, considerations for image enhancement, archiving, and photography pitfalls are discussed.

## 7.1  Equipment

Although cell phones are widely used by law enforcement for informal photography, a cell phone camera is not sufficient for scientific or comprehensive crime scene documentation. Also, there are ethical concerns that come into play when taking, storing, or sharing images of decedents (in whatever state) from a cell phone. A camera kit, with dedicated high quality equipment, is essential. This kit should be used in the laboratory and at the crime scene, and should include the items listed in Table 7.1.

There are many excellent references on forensic photography that include in-depth discussions of shutter speed, aperture, ISO (standardized sensitivity of the camera sensors to light) and specific lighting (Mancini and Sidoriak 2017; Marsh 2014; Robinson 2016; Weiss 2008) and thus a full discussion of the mechanics of photography will not be included here.

A camera with exceptional resolution will have large file sizes to match. The laboratory infrastructure must be able to handle photographs with dedicated image processing software and a computer powerful enough to hold and process the images in a timely manner. Digital storage capacity is also required.

## 7.2  Taking photographs with an eye to courtroom presentation

Basic forensic photographic training is essential to be a successful forensic practitioner and is one of the most under-trained areas in Forensic Anthropology

(1) Ample photographs critical to document scene prior to/during processing.

(2) Remove tools and personnel from photographs.

(3) Take care to avoid shadows (esp. camera operator) in photographs.

(4) Ensure that photographs depict everything observed: scene and laboratory.

(5) Photographs should be overlapping and sequential.

(6) Each photograph must be able to stand on its own in legal proceedings.

(7) Check digital images for clarity and efficacy; do they depict observation?

(8) Original, unaltered images must be maintained for every case.

**Figure 7.1** Forensic photography points to remember.

(Figure 7.1). A good forensic photograph is composed with relevant information, sufficient context to provide understanding, has proper exposure, and is in sharp focus on the critical areas. Forensic photography is not artistic photography, differing in purpose and production.

Like all data and documents associated with case work, laboratory standard operating procedures (SOPs) should include information on how photographs should be taken, filed, stored, and retained by the agency. Access to different storage media change with time and SOPs should be regularly updated to reflect changing technology. Good overall photographs of the scene, comprehensive and logically taken, will help preserve the integrity of the crime scene and evidence. In taking these photographs, consideration of the audience (law enforcement, coroners, medical examiners, attorneys, other experts) is important. The photographs should follow a logical progression, overlap when appropriate and not jump from place to place. The mechanics of crime scene and laboratory documentation basically follow a formula of overall, midrange and close up (with and without a scale) images. Care should be taken so that photographs separated from the sequence still contain the information necessary to understand the context. Many times, single photographs are admitted into evidence through the Forensic Anthropologist and they must be able to stand on their own. This point is crucial and cannot be overstated.

Whenever possible, exclude recovery team members and other personnel and their equipment from the photographs. People and tools are distracting in an image that may, one day, find itself in the courtroom. The exception to this rule is when their work is the reason the photograph is being taken, for example documenting the extraction of remains from an awkward situation or when the people are re-enacting how a body may have been handled in order to be deposited at the site originally. Typically, focusing on the decedent and the scene, rather than the distraction of personnel or tools, transmits a stronger sense of professionalism and respect to the jury.

At the crime scene, photographs should be taken as a sequence in a logical manner so that a viewer, and ultimately the jury, has the experience of moving through the scene. Crime scene specialists sometimes refer to this as "four-cornering a room." The concept is to photograph the entire room from each corner so that everything is documented. A good photographer will extend the idea to outdoor scenes and to documentation of the decedent.

In complex scenes, a "bulls-eye" approach is helpful where the area of interest is central to the overall, midrange and close-up images (Figure 7.2). Overall photographs depict large portions of the crime scene or an overall photograph of the remains (Figure 7.2a). They show the surrounding environment and the areas where access is possible and not possible. They often show how visible the scene would be to others in the area.

Midrange photographs depict the relationships between smaller components of the scene, allowing the fine detail of a smaller portion of items to be viewed (Figure 7.2b). Like overall photographs, they should be logically sequenced, often after an overall photograph is taken so that the context of the midrange photograph is understood.

Finally, close-up photos (with and without a scale) show specific orientation, condition, and characteristics of an item (Figure 7.2c). Close-up photos may also be used for examination and comparison. As such, overall and midrange photographs are primarily used to establish the context of the item in the close-up photo. In order to use a photograph for comparison purposes or examination in general, a scale is placed on the same plane as the defect. Photographs are taken with the lens at a right angle to the object or area of interest to limit distortion due to different focal lengths and camera angles. Having the scale in the same plane as the defect and with the photograph taken at a right angle to the defect, the image can be scaled 1 : 1 and effectively used as a reference for comparison and examination.

Filling the frame of the photograph ensures that each pixel is dedicated to the image being recorded rather than being wasted on extraneous material. This approach will have a significant impact later when enlarging images to extract detail or when they are projected on a large screen in the courtroom. However, high resolution does not make up for poor composition or excessive distance from the object being photographed. Either physically getting closer to the object or scene or using a lens that will provide appropriate magnification is the approach to take in order to maximize utilization of the frame.

In photography, the size of the aperture (f-stop), shutter speed and sensitivity of the camera sensor to light (ISO) are linked to control lighting and depth

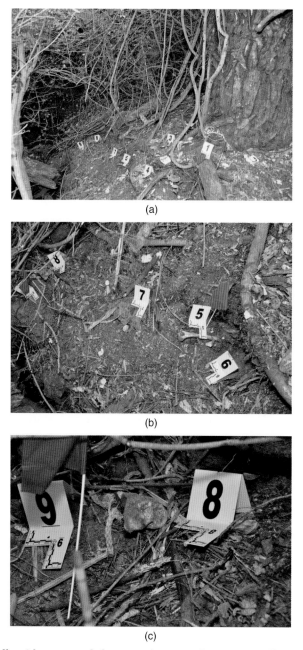

(a)

(b)

(c)

**Figure 7.2** Overall, midrange, and close-up photographs. (a) Overall photograph showing the relationship amongst a large area and multiple items. (b) Midrange photo depicting the relationship and details of a smaller group of items. (c) Close-up photo of item 8. The proximal end of a partially buried tibia and rope are visible in the center of the photo (bullseye). This detail is not clearly visible in the overall or midrange photo.

of field and can be utilized to clarify the purpose of the photograph. There are situations where special lighting techniques or blurring of a background may help document specific features of the case. However, sharp focus of the main item of interest is critical. Understanding depth of field (the area that will be in focus) is important. Depth of field is dependent on the size of the aperture (size of the opening in the diaphragm of the lens), which on a camera is measured using the f-stop. Use of a large aperture, for example f/2.8, will minimize the area of focus and blur other parts of the image, while use of a smaller aperture, such as f/11, will increase the distances from the camera that are in focus in the photograph. In forensic photography, adjusting aperture can be used to highlight specific details by keeping the depth of field tight, or provide context for an observation by increasing the depth of field, which is best for general crime scene photography. For example, with a large aperture, a single bone within a skeleton may be in sharp focus but with a small aperture and longer time of exposure, the entire skeleton will be in focus. The ability to control depth of field is a compelling reason to take the camera off "auto" and manually control the aperture and length of exposure. Thinking about how the image may be used in a report or in court is critical to this decision.

As aperture, shutter speed and ISO are linked, increasing or decreasing the size of the aperture will reduce or increase the amount of light let in to the camera for a given shutter speed. ISO can assist as the third variable to control the amount of light because it monitors how rapidly the camera can produce an image with the given amount of light. It is essentially equivalent to the "film speed" in non-digital cameras. When a high ISO is selected on the camera, the photograph can capture the image more quickly with a shorter time of exposure. However, the image will have more "noise," seen as increasing graininess of the image and the resulting artifacts affect the overall quality of the photo. A low ISO will produce a better image but require a longer time for the camera lens to be open.

Faster shutter speeds are needed when action shots are involved, so that the movement of people or objects do not result in blurring. This need is less likely the situation with forensic photography. Slower shutter speeds, however, may introduce perceivable camera shake and focus problems. When holding the camera in the hand, a good rule of thumb is to avoid using a shutter speed slower than 1/60th of a second. Any slower means the use of a tripod is essential.

In addition to the mechanics of the camera, distance of the camera from the object being photographed and/or the focal length of the lens is critical. Focal length determines the magnification of the image by the camera and the amount of area that is within the frame. Figure 7.3 illustrates the same subject with the same lighting using different focal lengths, ranging from 17 to 105 mm. The actual distance between the camera and the skull remained the same in all the photographs at 29 in. (approximately 74 cm). However, the use of different focal

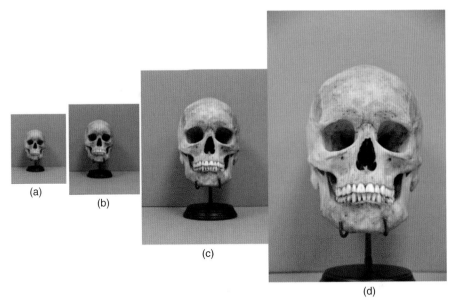

**Figure 7.3** Photos taken with different focal lengths: (a) 17 mm; (b) 24 mm; (c) 50 mm; and (d) 105 mm.

lengths can distort distances, an important consideration when trying to create a record of how a scene, bone, or other characteristic looked in "real life."

Additional lighting can be essential in forensic photography to allow for better focus and to illuminate the area or object of interest. Harsh lighting, however, is problematic with bone as it excessively lights the surface, resulting in overexposure of the area of interest, which will then appear as extremely white/yellow on the image. Use of diffusion filters over lights is helpful to reduce the overexposure, or manual adjustment of the flash power. Photography of highly reflective surfaces will be difficult with lighting as the camera will register the reflected light and mask other objects. Photographs with water or other reflective surfaces, as in photographs of a partially submerged body, may benefit from use of a polarizing filter over the lens, which will reduce glare but will require adjustments of aperture, shutter speed or ISO to achieve a properly exposed photo.

Placement of the lighting is another factor to be considered. Lighting at oblique angles reduces the potential for glare and may be useful to bring out detail not visible with direct lighting. Such lighting is particularly useful when highlighting surface texture or defects. Figure 7.4 illustrates the same pubic symphysis shot with a 60 mm lens with lighting at different angles. This series of pubis photographs was shot using a Nikon D800 camera with 60 mm macro lens with the aperture at F8. A detachable flash was used positioned at different angles to demonstrate the change in appearance of the pubic symphysis due

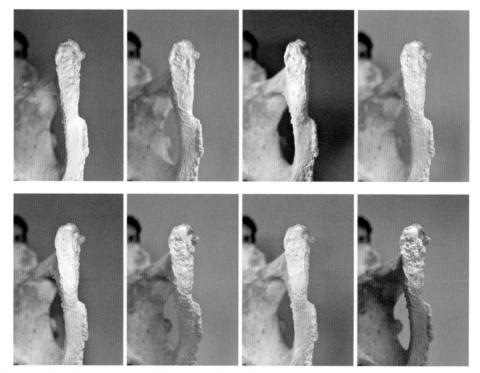

**Figure 7.4** Lighting used at different angles will accentuate different detail.

to lighting angle. In some cases, all surface detail on the joint surface is lost due to over-lighting while in others portions are visible but other areas are obscured. The final image (lower right corner) shows clear detail across the surface, sufficient to record the features used in age estimation.

In most cases, shadows are not the friend of the forensic photographer (Figure 7.5). Areas not lighted or lighted inappropriately may lead to missed evidence and a distorted view of the item. As a general rule, fill flash, leaving the flash on for indoor and outdoor photography, is recommended at all times. Additionally, the use of a detachable flash and not the camera's on-board flash is recommended, especially when using longer lenses. If the flash is not strong enough to light the subject, use of a longer lens will create the shadow of a half-moon in the photograph. Gaining a clear understanding of the equipment prior to first use, so that the photographer can capture what the human eye is seeing and how contrast and lighting will affect the final image, is critical.

Skeletal elements can be difficult to photograph when there is a sharp contrast between the bone and the background surface causing cameras to try to compensate for the difference. Photography on a black cloth will eliminate many of the background shadows but the contrast can confuse the camera sensors and often

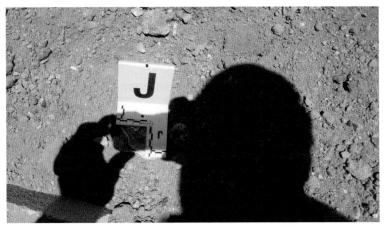

**Figure 7.5** Problematic photograph where contrast between shadow and intense light obscure the object in question. Having the shadow of the photographer in the photograph is unprofessional and can be avoided by moving to the other side of the object being photographed.  Source: Courtesy of SLOFIST.

leads to overexposure of the item being photographed. Use of gray or blue backgrounds often lowers the contrast and allows the image to be better calculated. Red backgrounds should be avoided since these images will potentially be used in court and red may be deemed too suggestive of violence.

To enable color correction of images, use of a white balance card or color chart is helpful in the post production for accurate images. The use of a color chart in the original photos is useful in court as well. Attorneys often receive photocopies of the photographs, rather than actual images and the color can be altered significantly by the copier used. Trying to demonstrate subtle color changes, particularly in trauma cases, becomes extremely frustrating when the color does not accurately represent the specimen being photographed.

Aside from focus, lighting and filling the frame, common pitfalls with forensic photography include incomplete documentation in the image so that it cannot be readily associated with a case number, insufficient photographs, and lack of photographs establishing context and odd angles. With digital cameras, caution warrants taking many photographs rather than too few. A scene cannot be recreated once it has been processed so careful, meticulous documentation is imperative.

## 7.3  Labeling photographs

There is a large variety of labeling equipment for use at the scene and in the laboratory. Images with and without associated scales are important. Perhaps the most important accessory is a placard, which can be very simple. Information that is important, particularly for a scene recovery is the case number, date, photographer and start and end times. Bracketing a series of images with a photograph of the case number at the beginning and end of each sequence allows for easy separation of material later. The bracketing placard photographs also ensures that future consumers of the images know they have all images that are available and in cases where there is an error in folder labeling, the placards can be used as a reference to make sure they are the correct images for the case. In addition, a photo log can be maintained when the Forensic Anthropologist is responsible for documenting the scene, and even in the laboratory.

## 7.4  Photomicroscopy and Videography

In some cases, photomicroscopy is important for documentation of details not visible, or difficult to visualize, with the naked eye (Figure 7.6). Most microscopes can be fitted with camera attachments, often relatively inexpensively. These photographs allow information such as cut mark contours, kerf floor profiles or

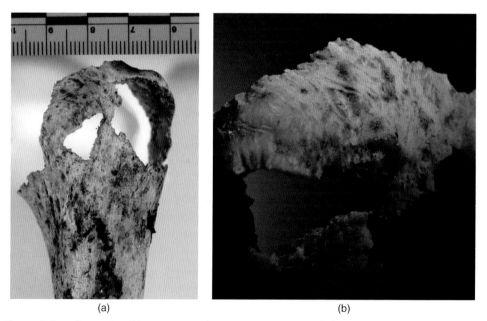

(a)                                                (b)

**Figure 7.6** Left proximal humerus with postmortem animal damage. (a) Midrange photo depicting the proximal end. Much of the proximal end is missing and what is present has a scooped-out appearance. (b) Photo taken using oblique lighting and a low powered stereo microscope. Notice how the detail in the striations is developed by light making the damage clearly attributable to rodent activity versus an antemortem pathological condition.

osteon and cementum annulation rings to be included in a report in a way that is verifiable by another viewer.

The use of video documentation can be extremely helpful in very complex crime scenes as a complement to still photography. Video works best when the audio is off unless it is possible for the associated personnel to discontinue work and remain silent. Sounds will be distracting for a jury or judge and are often taken as signs of disrespect by the family and friends of the decedent.

Begin and end each video with a shot of a placard showing the case number and date. Video quality is enhanced when the videographer moves and walks very slowly, much slower than one thinks necessary. Many departments have internal policies on the pattern of filming so some videos must be continuous while others can be stopped and started as needed. Video is particularly suited for documenting initial walk-throughs, crime scene processes, and final walk-throughs. It can also be useful, given current technology, of informing others who are remotely situated as to the information at the scene. This can also be useful in minimizing the personnel present at a scene as it is being processed.

## 7.5  Image processing

Images can be adapted for use in the case report through the use of image processing and adjustment. Computer programs are routinely used to rotate, crop, and refine photographs. However, there are some precautions. First, the modified copy must be saved separately from the original image and the original image should be retained as a separate file. Secondly, a history of any modification should be maintained, including the decisions made by the person altering the image and how it was stored.

Digital files are also altered by the condensation protocols used in files such as .jpg and .pdf. Basic familiarity with these alterations is essential to preserve quality of the image. Repeated "saves" to a file may corrupt the quality of a compressed image over time. For the best archiving of images, keeping original photographs in a non-compressed file format, such as .tif or raw, is recommended. The .tif and raw files, when saved and closed, do not lose information to adjust to a smaller file size.

With digital photography, there is the freedom to take a large number of images and, consequently, there are a number that are of low quality. The temptation is to simply delete these images but forensic protocol and laboratory policy often dictates the opposite – retain all images, regardless of quality.

More than one archival copy of photographs, including original and any modified images, should be stored and maintained in a separate location or in a secured Cloud service. Duplication ensures that if a disaster happens, such as a server explosion or meltdown, another copy is available in the archives. Considering the average number of photos required to fully document a crime scene and laboratory exam can total hundreds of images (or more) with the addition of modified images for the report, memory and storage requirements are a serious consideration. However, going to court with poor images or having to reveal that original images are no longer available is extremely detrimental to a legal case. The care demonstrated in the photographs is a reflection of the meticulousness used in the analysis.

## 7.6 Conclusion

Photographs should reflect the observations and conclusions drawn in the case report. They can be regularly incorporated into reports or provided separately. They are subject to subpoena regardless of which method is employed. Forensic Anthropologists who work in a Medical Examiner/Coroner office must follow the protocols established by their office, however they can ensure that the photographs are properly obtained, contain the necessary markers (case number, scale, N arrow, and pointer as necessary), and of sufficient quality. Complete records of all photographs associated with a case are also important at the time of discovery should a case head to trial. For someone reassessing the case, such as the pathologist or an anthropologist retained by opposing counsel, the photographs may be the first line of evidence upon which they depend rather than the report itself. Therefore, the photographs should be easily understandable in their own right. Photographs are also critical for the experienced anthropologist. In the early period of practice, every case is clearly remembered but in the later period the anthropologist often finds they must rely on notes and photographs to refresh their memories.

In almost all cases, the photographs taken during recovery and analysis are those that form the basis for the courtroom presentation. All photographs are subject to subpoena whether they are "lifted" from the copy of the report provided to the attorneys in preparation of the case or provided separately. Direct communication with the attorneys prior to court is critical as the anthropologist or their agency should have digital versions of all report photographs that will be of better resolution than enlargements of the printed images provided to attorneys. This will allow the Forensic Anthropologist to suggest those images that best reflect their observations or the conclusions they will testify to in Court.

# References

Mancini, K. and Sidoriak, J. (2017). *Fundamentals of Forensic Photography: Practical Techniques for Evidence Documentation on Location and in the Laboratory*. New York: Routledge.

Marsh, N. (2014). *Forensic Photography: A Practitioner's Guide*. Hoboken, NJ: Wiley-Blackwell.

Robinson, E.M. (2016). *Crime Scene Photography*, 3e. Amsterdam: Academic Press.

Weiss, S.L. (2008). *Forensic Photography: Importance of Accuracy*. Upper Saddle River, NJ: Pearson/Prentice-Hall.

## CHAPTER 8

# The peer review process: expectations and responsibilities

Kristen Hartnett-McCann[1], Laura C. Fulginiti[2], Alison Galloway[3], and Katherine M. Taylor[4]

[1] State of Connecticut, Office of the Chief Medical Examiner, Farmington, CT, USA
[2] Maricopa County, Office of the Medical Examiner, Phoenix, AZ, USA
[3] University of California, Santa Cruz, Santa Cruz, CA, USA
[4] King County Office of the Medical Examiner, Seattle, WA, USA

## 8.1 Introduction

Much of the existing literature relating to scientific peer review focuses on peer review for research and publication, and not on scientific case reports. To fill the gap, this chapter focuses on the process of peer review and its legal implications relating to the final product of a forensic anthropological case examination: the Forensic Anthropology case report. Throughout this chapter, recommendations are provided that address the selection of peer reviewers, the expectations on the part of both reviewer and reviewee, how to mitigate the problems of bias within the peer review system as currently practiced, and the mechanics of how to document the process and results of such reviews.

The process of peer review is central to research, validation, and publication in scientific journals, and a publication that has successfully passed through peer review gains acceptance in the field. Furthermore, publication in a peer reviewed journal is an important consideration for admissibility of scientific evidence in courts of law (Kumar 2009), although judges may be less cognizant of its importance than desired (Kovera and McAuliff 2000). Peer review is the process by which written investigational findings from an author (or co-authors) are given to an individual or group of individuals (referees) in the field for assessment of their quality, accuracy, relevance, and novelty (Shuttleworth 2009). These reviews may be open in that all parties know the identities of the authors and reviewers, single blind in which case the authors do not know the identity of the reviewers or double blind in which neither party is informed as to the identity

*Forensic Anthropology and the United States Judicial System*, First Edition.
Edited by Laura C. Fulginiti, Kristen Hartnett-McCann, and Alison Galloway.
© 2019 John Wiley & Sons Ltd. Published 2019 by John Wiley & Sons Ltd.

of the other group. In general, the goals of peer review are to determine if an article or report is acceptable for publication, and to improve it through referee feedback (Neale and Bowman 2006).

The broader impacts of peer review have been extensively published (for examples see Bearinger 2006; Callaham and McCulloch 2011; Leek et al. 2011; Mayden 2012; McNutt et al. 1990; Smith 2006; van Rooyen et al. 1999). Peer review, in its ideal, provides constructive criticism on a body of writing and provides information on what can be done to improve the work. Often peer review is seen as a "gold standard" of the scientific community and a guarantor that the work is of the highest caliber.

Peer review has also been sharply criticized for failing to meet its primary objective of improving the quality of the manuscripts accepted for publication or validating the material in case reports (Ballantyne et al. 2017; Jefferson et al. 2002). Specifically, peer review can perform poorly in the face of confirmation bias and cognitive bias. The former is the tendency to accept the findings of another person with little significant challenge while the latter is the impact of prior knowledge on the conclusions drawn by the reviewer. In addition, there are also issues, at least in journal reviews, of longitudinal deterioration with the quality of reviews from individual reviewers (Callaham and McCulloch 2011).

## 8.2 Historical use of peer review

An historical perspective of peer review for Forensic Anthropology case reports does not exist because it is a relatively recent phenomenon which lacks a formal process. Peer review in the academic setting, however, has a history dating back to the mid-1700s when a group of scholars formed a commission to vet manuscripts submitted to the Royal Society of Edinburgh (Spier 2002). The concept was rooted in a quasi-censorship, however, in which the royally appointed academies and scholarly societies read material and approved that which was felt to reinforce the reputation and royal support of the society (Biagioli 2002; Ranalli 2011). By the mid-1800s, peer review had begun to gain wider traction because journals were expected to invest primarily in articles that produced new data or interpretations, and that were scientifically rigorous. In order to make this selection, peer review was adopted, usually as a single blind process. At the time, politics and scientific in-fighting were readily displayed in such a process. The reviewers were called upon to defend the reputation of the journal by only accepting worthy publications but were able to also affect the careers, positively and negatively, of those they reviewed. By the late 1800s, the flow of scholarly works had grown to the point that peer review was also seen as a way of reducing the influx of manuscripts to a manageable level, selecting only those manuscripts that would have the greatest impact on the discipline.

By the mid-1990s, a double blind process was gaining wider application in journal reviews. In double blind reviews, the file to be reviewed is stripped of any indication of authorship (such as author names and institutional affiliations) so the work must be judged on the merits of the product alone, and the reviewer is not known to the author. Today, in traditional research-based publications as well as in granting agencies, the peer review process is ideally conducted "in the blind" (double blind review). However, in small communities, the origin of papers is still often apparent due to clues in the approach, topic, or location of the fieldwork. The use of a separate statistical review (a checklist of specifics that are used to quantify a review) has also gained ground. Blind reviews do not appear to adversely affect or benefit the quality of the review above the influence of an editor, although if the reviewer is to be identified to the author, more reviewers decline to review (van Rooyen et al. 1999).

With the advent of online submission and publication, journals may also use a completely open system (Smith 2006). In this application of peer review, the manuscript is posted along with any solicited reviews but all are available for open comment from the community. This type of review is not suitable for the Forensic Anthropology case report but may be a useful format for scientific works in that the strengths and weaknesses of any methodology that is published is then available to both prosecution and defense (Jones 2007). The benefits of this approach have not yet been fully evaluated.

Conscious or unconscious bias is a common problem in peer reviews due to the subjective nature of the process. Historically, bias played a major role in who was accepted and who was rejected. Studies have shown that significant bias against women and against those who are employed at less prestigious institutions have plagued peer review for journals and granting agencies (Peters and Ceci 1982; Wennarås and Wold 1997). The bias may also be more personal in nature, where the work of rivals may be sharply criticized or even stolen (Smith 2006).

## 8.3   Principles underlying peer review in Forensic Anthropology

In Forensic Anthropology, peer review exists in two critical positions. One, as is most commonly understood within the academic community, is in the peer review of research prior to publication. Once a manuscript is submitted to a journal for consideration, the work is sent by the journal editors to outside and independent researchers who evaluate the validity of the research as well as the soundness of the findings. These reviewers will also assess the clarity of the communication, its appropriateness in the journal to which it has been submitted, and its significance to the broader community. This type of peer review for published works is critical in the assessment of the worthiness of the research prior to admission in court under applicable rules of evidence (see Chapters 1 and 2).

In the second application of peer review in Forensic Anthropology, case reports are assessed by another Forensic Anthropologist prior to submission to the agency requesting the service. Case report peer review is growing rapidly with the increase in accreditation and published standards of practice. Such reviews involve a check on the basic structure, usually called an administrative review (correct labels, typographic errors, alignment of figures to citations in text, etc.), and a deeper assessment of the appropriateness of the methodologies used and the validity of the findings and interpretations, usually called a technical review. Finally, the clarity of the entire report (text and images) is addressed.

The case report (see Chapter 6) forms the basis for the Forensic Anthropologist's court testimony. This document is exchanged between counsels prior to the appearance of the expert and should reflect the bulk of the information that will be presented in court. Ensuring that written work, in this case the written case report, is sound and clearly written prior to submission allows for both prosecution and defense, or plaintiff and defendant, to understand and prepare for the direct and cross examinations, provides the defendant (and counsel) with a reasonable assessment of what they can present in rebuttal, and prevents delays in the trial due to "surprise" testimony.

## 8.4   Available guidance on peer review

Currently, there are no professionally endorsed standards in Forensic Anthropology for the application of methods regarding the recovery, analysis, and documentation of human remains. Similarly, there are no standards for peer review. Instead, we have to look to a series of sources that focus on quality management within the discipline. Overall, there are three interconnected sources of information: (i) SWGANTH (Scientific Working Group in Anthropology), (ii) NIST/OSAC (National Institute of Science and Technology/Organization of Scientific Area Committees), and (iii) accreditation standards in forensic sciences.

The SWGANTH documents, drafted through the collaborative effort of Forensic Anthropologists under the support of the Federal Bureau of Investigation (FBI) and the Department of Defense beginning formally in 2008, were the first effort to provide more broadly applicable standards. The only SWGANTH document that mentions peer review is the Laboratory Management and Quality Assurance document, and in it peer review is called "technical review." According to this document, a laboratory should have policies and procedures in place for external and/or internal technical review (evaluation of a test and/or report and associated supporting documentation) and administrative reviews (focusing on editorial correctness). In many cases, these two reviews are combined into one (SWGANTH 2011).

The SWGANTH documents form the foundation of the standards, guidelines, and best practice recommendations that the US NIST is drafting for OSAC approval. As of 2018, none of these documents have reached the level of OSAC approval. Within the available drafts, there are no agreed-upon guidelines as to who is a qualified peer reviewer, and there are no overarching guidelines or standards for how to perform a peer review of a Forensic Anthropology case report.

Some individual agencies or institutions, as well as sole practitioners, have developed their own case report peer review rubrics based on various accreditation guidelines, or have adopted guidelines from other disciplines. Larger organizations, such as the Defense POW/MIA Accounting Agency (DPAA) and FBI, and some large Medical Examiner Offices, are accredited by accrediting bodies (e.g. the National Association of Medical Examiners). In addition, the ANSI-ASQ National Accreditation Board (ANAB) is a US-based non-governmental organization that provides ISO (International Organization for Standardization) accreditation services, such as ISO/IEC 17020 (2012) and ISO/IEC 17025 (2005). Using these guidelines, laboratories have written their standard operating procedures (SOPs) including some sections on peer review (see Chapter 5).

While none of these approaches provide specific requirements or templates for peer review in Forensic Anthropology, they do provide some insight into the probable expectations of the peer review process in the future. Overall, the language in the ISO/IEC documents (ISO/IEC 17020 and 17025) is generalized in order for it to apply to all fields. An accrediting body will usually expect the applicant organization to address the following: (i) is there a peer review process in place, (ii) is it recorded in the case file, (iii) does it allow for results/observations to be rejected, (iv) is there a process in place for how to proceed if there is non-concurrence, (v) is the procedure written in the SOP, (vi) are qualified individuals performing the peer reviews, (vii) is there a method used for demonstrating the completion of each review (such as a checklist), (viii) is there an annual Management Review which includes all records that required a resolution, and (ix) does the peer review form show the name and signature of the person who is validating the case report? Future SOPs, standards, and best practice recommendations for peer review may be expected to fall in line with the ISO/IEC 17020 and/or 17025 standards, both of which significantly overlap in their peer review content.

While the information on peer review is somewhat sparse in these documents discussed above, the practitioner or agency/laboratory is responsible for following the best practice recommendations and guidelines and expanding upon these recommendations in SOPs or other laboratory guidelines. In an example of how this guidance is enacted, the FBI Laboratory recently made all of its quality assurance documents available online (http://www.fbilabqsd.com). The FBI Laboratory Operations manual provides a small amount of information on Administrative Reviews and Technical Reviews. According to their Operations manual, Administrative Review ensures that the record is complete, uses correct spelling and grammar, is properly classified, and complies with FBI Laboratory Requirements and Practices. A Technical Review evaluates notes, data, and other supporting records that form the basis of the scientific results and conclusions contained in the report. The technical review consists of determining whether the appropriate examinations have been performed, the conclusions are consistent with the recorded data, and are within the scope of the discipline and/or category of testing (FBI Laboratory 2017).

In another example, specifically directed for work with skeletal material, the DPAA laboratory in Hawaii has an entire section of their SOPs (section 4.1; 7 pages long) devoted to the procedures used for internal and external peer review of all field/technical notes and reports. The DPAA utilizes mostly ISO/IEC 17025, although there are some issues addressed pertaining to ISO/IEC 17020.

## 8.5 Considerations

In our experience, peer review is an invaluable asset to improving the quality of reports from both the technical and administrative aspects as well as the scientific aspects. Peer review does not typically cost the reviewee anything, in terms of money, which eliminates the complicated involvement of agency finances. The process of peer review is not a way for reviewers to earn money or supplement their salary; more, it is a professional responsibility that we all have to each other in our discipline for both case report and publication peer reviews. That being said, the fact that an expert reviewer does not get paid for their expertise could also be seen as a negative (see Chapter 12).

Unlike peer review for research where the publication solicits and chooses peer reviewers, or in a large agency where an in-house peer reviewer is always assigned by a supervisor, a sole practitioner is the one who asks for and chooses the peer reviewer. The choice of who to ask to perform a peer review is difficult in that there are different criteria based on availability, willingness to do the review, reciprocity, and potential cost (time spent away from other duties) for the reviewer. The ideal person is someone with sufficient experience as both a Forensic Anthropologist as well as an expert witness in the courtroom to assess the report in terms of its accuracy within the discipline and its ability to communicate the findings to both professionals and a lay audience. In cases of homicide, the reviewer should be assessing the report in terms of what questions could be generated under cross-examination that would expose the original anthropologist to impeachment and to ensure that they have been answered in the report. For example, there may be alternative mechanisms that could produce a perimortem defect that should be addressed in the report or in the bench notes. The reviewer might, in this case, request that the report or bench notes reflect other possible interpretations. Overall, it is important that the report reflects the potential conclusions from the evidence, and that the reviewing Forensic Anthropologist can reach the same conclusions as those in the original report.

The benefits of peer review for case reports are offset by some more problematic aspects, and these are often cited as reasons why all case reports are not peer reviewed. Peer review is a time-consuming process, increasing the time needed to complete and file a case, and can be subject to reviewer availability. Typically, it can easily add an additional week to the time needed to complete the report if the reviewer is not available in-house. Furthermore, some Forensic Anthropologists may see peer review as a burden, especially if they are reviewing outside their normal employment. There is always a possibility that the reviewer might be subpoenaed for court testimony and could have to travel to meet that obligation.

All reviewers are subject to bias, whether it be gender, age, institution, nationality, status in the field, linguistic preferences, or writing style/ability. Reviewers should disclose any known biases that may prevent an impartial review. In addition, reviewers should inform the reviewee if there is a lack of expertise in a particular relevant area which may hinder the review.

The use of in-house reviewers can also be questioned as to their independence and training experience. That both parties are employed by the same agency may create underlying bias and there are difficulties in isolating exposure to a case by those in the same discipline working within one facility. Likewise, if the two individuals are trained by the same person, or if one trained the other, then there will be training bias in the review. In the latter situation and in a tiered position laboratory, there are supervisory or evaluative lines involved between the reviewer and reviewee that can hinder an independent assessment, even without overt pressure.

Finally, peer review can also fail, allowing fraudulent or sub-par reports to be finalized. This failure may occur when the peer review process is not taken as a serious commitment but a "rubber stamp" for a colleague. There could be failure because of an unwillingness to call-out a colleague or friend when disagreements occur, or when the reviewer is not well-prepared to evaluate current methods or assessments.

## 8.6   Current status of peer review in forensic anthropological casework

In order to assess the current utilization of peer review in forensic anthropological case work, a survey was distributed to the Anthropology Section of the American Academy of Forensic Sciences in 2018. Fifty-seven responses were received with slightly over half reporting that they participate in peer review for all their cases. A further 17.9% participate for 75–99% of cases, usually excluding those of non-human material or archeological context. In all, almost 70% use peer review for their cases of forensic significance. Less than 10% do not submit cases for peer review at all. Of the 57 respondents, approximately 68% use a reviewer from the same office or agency, while 21% use a reviewer from an outside agency or office.

Less common were agency policies for peer review that follow an accepted standard or guideline, such as ISO/IEC 17020. Only 32.1% of respondents reported having such agency policies in place while 44.6% did not. Almost one-quarter of respondents were not sure whether there were or were not policies. The independent responses tended to list ISO/IEC 17020 or 17025 as the most commonly used reference, although in-house SOPs were also cited.

Responses were almost evenly divided regarding inclusion of peer review within the SOPs of individual labs. Half reported that peer review was not included in the SOP while the remainder said that it was (46.4%) or they were not sure (3.6%). When asked if there were peer review forms that accompanied the SOPs, slightly more than half (52.6%) responded that there were.

When asked about the frequency at which reviews are conducted, responses were quite mixed. The vast majority (74.5%) reported only writing 25 or less case report peer reviews in a year. This percentage was about evenly divided between those writing less than 5 and those writing between 5 and 25 reviews. The majority (63%) maintain records of their reviews, usually on a spreadsheet.

Respondents were asked if they have ever been questioned about peer review during court testimony. Only 33 respondents had testified based on their case reports, and of those, approximately 20% have been asked about peer review. Two-thirds were not asked about peer review by the attorneys during testimony, a number that is likely to change in coming years. Only one respondent reported having been asked on the stand about a case for which they provided peer review.

In order to gauge the direction of peer reviewed material, we asked about how many cases and which types of cases *should* be reviewed. Over 60% stated that all cases should undergo a peer review process, and no one thought that peer review should be avoided completely. Almost all agreed that human cases of forensic significance should be peer reviewed around biological profile, trauma, postmortem interval and identification. There was slightly less insistence around reviews for pathological or anomalous conditions and scene response reports. One respondent also added that international cases (dealing with mass graves and human rights violations) should always be peer reviewed.

Over 60% of individual respondents did report participating in an informal or unofficial peer review process whereby case materials including photographs, bench notes, checklists, report drafts, and other information are shared for a "second opinion." This process was separate from the official process of peer review and is not usually included in the case file. The informal peer review can also be viewed as a bridge to a more formal peer review. One would start by seeking a second opinion on a certain aspect of a case, which would then open the door to a more formal review of the entire case report.

## 8.7   Recommendations on peer review of forensic anthropology case work

Formal peer review for every Forensic Anthropology report is ideal. Many practitioners do not have the time or resources to solicit peer review for all of their caseloads, some of which number in the hundreds annually. Likewise, within the discipline there are insufficient networks and resources for routine peer review, be it formal or informal. There are a small number of board-certified individuals and not all practitioners are experienced in trauma analyses and period since death; these are two of the common areas involving expert testimony. Since there is tremendous regional variability for time since death, peer review may be more challenging. While informal peer review does not require the documentation of a more formal process it can still add valuable critique. Each Forensic Anthropologist should strive to obtain formal peer review for as many of their forensic case reports as possible. Cases that may become involved in the legal process, complex trauma interpretation, and all infant/child evaluations should undergo peer review.

Peer review can be time consuming and difficult; therefore, accepting the responsibility of peer review requires commitment on the part of the reviewer. The process should be viewed as a professional responsibility, given that the end result can contribute to a cause and manner of death, an identification, and may ultimately end up in a court of law. Reviewers should respect the report author and the Forensic Anthropology report process, producing a quality of work that both are willing to stand behind, and that meets the best practices in the field.

Peer review does *not* shift the burden of responsibility for the scientific findings from the analyst to the reviewer.

A peer reviewer should be an experienced Forensic Anthropologist with complex analytical skills, which allows for the critical analysis of the report. In some agencies, only competency and proficiency tested Forensic Anthropologists can perform peer reviews. Peer reviews should never be conducted by the report author(s) and peer reviewers should have no immediate involvement with the case being reviewed. In addition, to protect the integrity of the peer review process, practitioners should seek out various individuals to perform peer reviews and not rely on one person for all reviews. In other words, one person should not be the sole, habitual reviewer of another's work.

Any peer review should be structured so that the author of the report must answer to the review itself (and not be able to just ignore it if they do not like it). The case report author must be held accountable and ways to mitigate negative reviews must be established. Cooperation between the author and reviewer is a factor that is positively associated with increased accuracy of the process (Leek et al. 2011) and should be encouraged. To achieve this level of cooperation, both parties must understand the gravity of a peer review of case reports and case files. The author must be aware that they are soliciting and will seriously consider any feedback from the reviewer.

As illustrated above, approximately 68% of the survey respondents use a peer reviewer from the same office or agency, while 21% use a reviewer from an outside agency or office. For those individuals with in-house peer review, the process is usually dictated by SOPs for the laboratory or other standards that are followed (such as ISO/IEC 17020 or 17025). Many Forensic Anthropologists, however, are sole practitioners. Ideally, the development of a remote peer review system or network for sole practitioners for soliciting peer reviews would be beneficial to our field. Since we do not (yet) have such a network available in our field, Forensic Anthropologists must seek out colleagues, former mentors, or former students who are willing and qualified to do peer reviews. In some agencies, there may be strict confidentiality rules (such as the Health Insurance Portability and Accountability Act, HIPAA) which would prohibit an external review. In these cases, a Forensic Anthropologist may have to rely on another in-house professional, such as a pathologist or odontologist, to perform a peer review. In some instances, these reviews may be more appropriate given the content of the report. Even with these challenges, our discipline should strive to incorporate peer review as a standard practice in forensic anthropological case work.

The usual modality for requesting formal and informal external peer reviews among colleagues is email or other electronic communication. Once an invitation to review a case report is accepted, reviewers normally agree to complete the report review within a specified time frame. Time is especially important in high profile cases or cases where a quick turn-around is needed by the agency for missing persons searches or legal matters. The peer review should be completed within one week from the receipt of the documents for external reviews, and within three business days for internal reviews. Case reports, bench notes, select photographs, and select diagrams are usually shared digitally, via email or other document sharing websites. The document sharing modalities must be trustworthy and the reviewer must maintain confidentiality throughout the process; using any information gained for self-interest or teaching is unethical. Keep in mind that emails are also subject to public records requests, which may be a problem especially in high profile cases. Agencies may require an official Memorandum of Understanding (MOU) between a reviewee and reviewer before these confidential materials can be shared. These MOUs are usually drafted by a legal department affiliated with an agency or institution, and which both parties sign prior to the peer review. Informal peer reviews, which are an unofficial sharing of documents or images for a "second opinion," are a mutual understanding between individuals and are not documented in writing or included in the case file.

Prior to conducting the review, the reviewer should ascertain what the expectations were of the Forensic Anthropologist who wrote the report (i.e. is the analysis solely on trauma and time since death since an identification had already been made?). Similarly, the requesting anthropologist should blind the report and associated documentation from any known information about the case. A peer reviewer who is aware of the known information will more likely accept rather than challenge the interpretation of the original analyst. During the review, comments and suggested revisions should be recorded in the body of the text of the report, in the report margins, and on the peer review form (if provided) in permanent media (i.e. no pencil). Stick on notes, scrap paper, and verbal comments should not be used. Grammar is important, and errors/typos should be pointed out; however, the main concerns for the reviewer are that the report author(s) addressed the requested analyses, the data in the bench notes and photographs match the report, that valid and appropriate methods are used, and that the conclusions are sound. Table 8.1 illustrates some suggested components of a typical peer review.

Typical peer reviews do not involve a full physical retesting of the all of the evidence, but if possible, "spot checks" of certain sections, such as measurements, assessing characteristics for the biological profile, or viewing questionable defects are highly recommended for in-house reviewers or those with access to the remains. For those reviewers who do not have direct access to the remains, the review can only focus on what can be discerned from the images and provided documents.

**Table 8.1** Important questions to consider when reviewing a Forensic Anthropology case report.

| | |
|---|---|
| Do you concur with the overall findings? | Are there any areas that could benefit from further explanation or analysis? |
| Does the report present relevant conclusions related to the examined cases(s)? | Is the report structured and formatted properly? |
| Are the results and conclusions presented accurate and evidence based? | If appropriate, are references provided in the report or notes, and what is the quality of the references? |
| Are the results and conclusions presented based on valid and appropriate methods/techniques? | If appropriate, are the photographs and diagrams clear and labeled? |
| Do the bench notes and photographs match the conclusions in the report? | Are there any areas in the report that should be deleted or relegated to the bench notes? |
| Do the case numbers on each page of the report and notes match? | Is there any information in the bench notes that should be included in the report? |
| Is the writing clear and concise? | Are there any ethical concerns or bias? |

Once the review is finished, the reviewer will complete a peer review form (which is usually provided by the reviewee), or will communicate specific comments in another format to the reviewee. The reviewer should comment on whether or not they concur with the overall findings in the report as a whole, and then provide input on each specific section (Figure 8.1).

Feedback should be professional and constructive. The length of the review is not as important as detailed comments or suggestions. If a reviewer feels that they cannot adequately evaluate a case based on the evidence provided, they may request additional materials (such as more photographs or diagrams). A report may be reviewed more than one time, depending on the degree of concurrence, and the number of times it is reviewed is subject to the discretion of the peer reviewer or in some cases, a Laboratory Director or Supervisor/Manager. Overall, the reviewer should offer scholarly input with the intent to improve the report and to ultimately concur with the findings. The peer review must be signed and dated by all reviewers. Again, there are no universally available peer review forms. These forms can be very brief, and consist only of a blank page to be filled in with comments, or they can be quite an extensive checklist with subheadings for every possible aspect of a Forensic Anthropology case report. Two examples of a peer review form are included in Appendices 8.A. and 8.B.

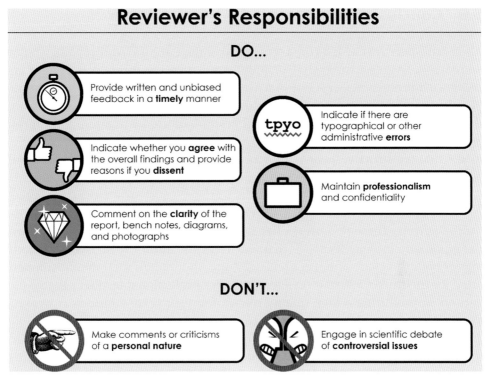

**Figure 8.1** Reviewer's responsibilities in Forensic Anthropology report peer reviews.

Upon return of the review, the reviewee should address or acknowledge each substantive (non-editorial) comment, suggestion, or recommendation by checking or initialing the comments on the sheet or in the text of the draft report. The reviewee should indicate agreement or disagreement with each comment, suggestion, or recommendation and what action was taken, if appropriate. Often the reviewer will withhold signing the peer review form until they see the revised version of the report and can validate that all comments were addressed, and the altered wording is consistent with their expectations – and that no new errors have been introduced. The reviewer may alter their original objection upon further explanation or documentation from the original report writer.

When disagreements arise between the reviewer/reviewee, appropriate measures should be taken to mitigate the problems. In some agencies, a higher level of review at the management or supervisor level may be needed to arbitrate the differences. For independent analysts, seeking a second reviewer may be necessary. In the end, the completed form should be retained in the case file.

## 8.8  Conclusions

A scientific peer review is a core component of the Forensic Anthropology report and case file, which ensures that all findings and methods meet an acceptable and recognized professional level of practice. Even though peer review is currently ill-defined and is not universally practiced in our field, it is still a gold standard that will continue to drive scholarly publication and serve as a tool for improving Forensic Anthropology case reports. The responsibility lies with the discipline to see that constructive peer review is included in future Forensic Anthropology standards, guidelines, or best practice recommendations, and that Forensic Anthropologists continue to maximize its use.

A large part of the success or failure of the peer review system rests with the peer reviewers. These reviewers offer scholarly input with the intent to improve the report and provide feedback that will allow the author to address shortcomings or points of confusion. Peer reviewers are, more often than not, uncompensated for their time. When a reviewer provides professional feedback that assists authors in producing a high quality report, the peer review process is working as intended. Reviewing also provides an opportunity for learning and gaining exposure to new methods or techniques for both parties. Although the peer review process can be lengthy and underappreciated, rewards such as learning, mentorship, exposure to new methods, and professional development make it a worthwhile endeavor. Peer review is a professional privilege and responsibility that directly impacts the quality of Forensic Anthropology in research, laboratory analyses, and ultimately, in the courtroom.

## Acknowledgments

We would like to thank the following individuals for their assistance with this chapter: Bradley Adams, Dana Austin, Angi Christensen, Gary Hodges, Jennifer Love, the Honorable Daniel Martin, Marin Pilloud, Vincent Sava, Caitlin Schrein, Angela Soler, and the 57 anonymous survey respondents.

## 8.A   Example of a peer review form (modified from Dana Austin, personal communication)

**PEER REVIEW FORM**

**(Your institution here)**

Date:_____          Case #:_____

Analyst: _____          Reviewer: _____

Circle N/A or Initial Applicable Statements

   ____   I <u>CONCUR</u> WITH THE FINDINGS

   ____   I <u>DO NOT CONCUR</u> WITH THE FINDINGS**
     *\*\*for situations of "non-concurrence," reviewer must include comments below*

**N/A**   ____   Reviewed all exhibits that the primary examiner is offering an opinion on.

**N/A**   ____   Reviewed the case file for supporting technical data, notes, and/or completed worksheets.

**N/A**   ____   Requested examinations have been addressed appropriately.

**N/A**   ____   Results are sound and reasonable, are clearly communicated, and were reached using accepted techniques by peers within this discipline

**N/A**   ____   Reviewed the case file for case numbers, required initials, and other errors.

Additional Comments:
_____

**Reviewer:**


_____          _____
Signature                                      Date

## 8.B Example of a peer review form (modified from Lauren Zephro, personal communication)

Peer Review Form

Case Agency and Number:

Reviewer:

Author of Report:

Date Materials Reviewed:

Description of the Material reviewed (# of pages of report, # of photographs, bench notes, casts, etc.):

Technical Review (correct technique, proper application, appropriate interpretations, supported conclusions):

Report Review (clarity of report and supporting information):

Additional comments:

By signing below, the Reviewer indicates that he/she finds the report and technical notes provided to them by the report's author satisfactory. If any portion of the submitted material was found to be unsatisfactory, the Reviewer has contacted the report's author and provided them an opportunity to clarify or amend the portion(s) in question.

Reviewer Signature: _____

Date of Review: _____

## References

Ballantyne, K.N., Edmond, G., and Round, B. (2017). Peer review in forensic science. *Forensic Science International* 277: 66–76.

Bearinger, L.H. (2006). Beyond objective and balanced: writing constructive manuscript reviews. *Research in Nursing & Health* 29: 71–73.

Biagioli, M. (2002). From book censorship to academic peer review. *Emergences* 12 (1): 11–45.

Callaham, M. and McCulloch, C. (2011). Longitudinal trends in the performance of scientific peer reviewers. *Annals of Emergency Medicine* 57: 141–148.

FBI Laboratory (2017). FBI Laboratory Operations Manual Definitions. Issue Date: 10/02/2017. Revision: 9. http://www.fbilabqsd.com. (accessed June 19, 2018).

ISO/IEC 17020. (2012). *Conformity assessment – Requirements for the operation of various types of bodies performing inspection*. Geneva: International Organization for Standardization/International Electrotechnical Commission.

ISO/IEC 17025. (2005). *General requirements for the competence of testing and calibration laboratories* (2e). Geneva: International Organization for Standardization/International Electrotechnical Commission.

Jefferson, T., Alderson, P., Wager, E., and Davidoff, F. (2002). Effects of editorial peer review: a systematic review. *Journal of the American Medical Association* 287 (21): 2784–2786.

Jones, A.W. (2007). The distribution of forensic journals, reflections on authorship practices, peer-review and role of the impact factor. *Forensic Science International* 165: 115–128.

Kovera, M.B. and McAuliff, B.D. (2000). The effects of peer review and evidence quality on judge evaluations of psychological science: are judges effective gatekeepers? *Journal of Applied Psychology* 85 (4): 574–586.

Kumar, M. (2009). A review of the review process: manuscript peer-review in biomedical research. *Biology and Medicine* 1 (4): 1–16.

Leek, J.T., Taub, M.A., and Pineda, F.J. (2011). Cooperation between referees and authors increases peer review accuracy. *Public Library of Science Medicine* 6 (11): e26895.

Mayden, K.D. (2012). Peer review: Publication's gold standard. *Journal of the Advanced Practitioner in Oncology* 3 (2): 117–122.

McNutt, R.A., Evans, A.T., Fletcher, R.H., and Fletcher, S.W. (1990). The effects of blinding on the quality of peer review. A randomized trial. *Journal of the American Medical Association* 263 (10): 1371–1376.

Neale, A.V. and Bowman, M.A. (2006). Peer review process of the Journal of the American Board of Family Medicine. *The Journal of the American Board of Family Medicine* 19 (2): 209–210.

Peters, D. and Ceci, S. (1982). Peer-review practices of psychological journals: the fate of submitted articles, submitted again. *Behavioral and Brain Science* 5: 187–255.

Ranalli, G. (2011). A prehistory of peer review: religious blueprints from the Hartlib Circle. *Spontaneous Generations: A Journal for the History and Philosophy of Science* 5 (1): 12–18.

Scientific Working Group for Forensic Anthropology (SWGANTH) (2011). Laboratory Management and Quality Assurance document. Issue Date: 06/25/2011. Revision: 1. https://www.nist.gov/topics/forensic-science/anthropology-subcommittee (accessed June 21, 2018).

Shuttleworth, M. (2009). Peer review process. http://www.experiment-resources.com/peer-review-process.html (accessed June 20, 2018).

Smith, R. (2006). Peer review: a flawed process at the heart of science and journals. *Journal of the Royal Society of Medicine* 99 (4): 178–182.

Spier, R. (2002). The history of the peer-review process. *Trends in Biotechnology* 20 (8): 357–358.

Van Rooyen, S., Godlee, F., Evans, S. et al. (1999). Effect of open peer review on quality of reviews and on reviewers' recommendations: a randomized trial. *British Medical Journal* 319 (7175): 23–27.

Wennarås, C. and Wold, A. (1997). Sexism and nepotism in peer review. *Nature* 387: 341–343.

## CHAPTER 9

# The United States justice system and forensic anthropology: preparing for court

Daniel G. Martin[1] and Laura C. Fulginiti[2]

[1] Maricopa County, Phoenix, AZ, USA
[2] Maricopa County, Office of the Medical Examiner, Phoenix, AZ, USA

The importance of expert testimony in the United States justice system cannot be overstated, and Forensic Anthropologists often play a critical role in that system. Some Forensic Anthropologists testify often, others only on occasion. But regardless of the frequency, the goal remains the same – helping others (often a jury or judge) understand evidence or determine a fact in issue. While the basic proposition is simple to state, the process can be complicated. Proper preparation is essential for even the most experienced practitioner; for those who are new to the system, it is critical.

The goal of this chapter is to provide insight into the legal system from experienced practitioners who have appeared in court on many occasions, and from a judicial officer who has presided over many different cases in which experts have appeared as witnesses. The chapter begins with an overview of the court system in the United States, and the judicial process in general. Next, the chapter addresses specific stages in the process during which the Forensic Anthropologist may play a role, up through and including trial testimony, and offers practical advice for avoiding common pitfalls. The chapter concludes with a discussion of courtroom etiquette, and "do's" and "don'ts" for expert witnesses.

## 9.1 The United States court system

The United States court system is split between state courts and federal courts (Figure 9.1). In addition, many Native American communities operate

*Forensic Anthropology and the United States Judicial System*, First Edition.
Edited by Laura C. Fulginiti, Kristen Hartnett-McCann, and Alison Galloway.
© 2019 John Wiley & Sons Ltd. Published 2019 by John Wiley & Sons Ltd.

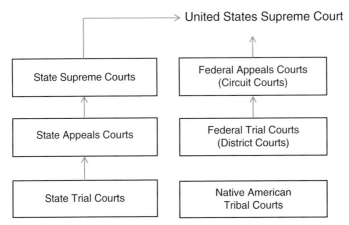

**Figure 9.1** The United States court system.

independent tribal courts. Within each of these systems, there are trial courts and there are appellate courts. While there are differences in names, all states have trial courts that hear a range of cases (typically civil, criminal, family, and juvenile). Some states call them superior courts, some call them circuit courts, and some call them courts of common pleas. But whatever the name, these are the courts in which the Forensic Anthropologist, as an expert witness, will most frequently appear, because these are the courts in which expert testimony is most often given.

Most states have an intermediate court of appeals, but in all states, the highest court is the Supreme Court. (In New York, the Supreme Court is the trial court, and the highest court is called the Court of Appeals, but that is not typical.) As a general rule, Forensic Anthropologists do not appear as experts in appeals courts, because those courts typically do not hold hearings or receive evidence; rather, they rely on the record created in the trial court.

In the federal system, the trial courts are called district courts. There is at least one district court in each state as well as the District of Columbia; some states have multiple districts (in California, for example, there are four districts). There are 94 district courts in all. The federal appeals courts are called circuit courts, and are divided into geographic regions. There are 13 circuit courts in total. The United States Supreme Court sits at the top of the federal court system, and by virtue of the Supremacy Clause of the United States Constitution (U.S. Constitution, article VI), the United States Supreme Court is also the final court of appeal for state court decisions that implicate constitutional and federal issues.

### 9.1.1   Types of cases

Both state and federal courts hear a number of different kinds of cases. At a very broad level, these cases fall within one of two categories – criminal and civil. In criminal cases, the government, whether state or federal, is prosecuting alleged violations of criminal laws. Civil cases are much broader in scope, and can involve any number of issues, from personal injury, to property disputes, to claims for breach of contract. Civil cases usually involve a dispute between individuals or entities. Sometimes one of those entities is the government, such as, for example, when the government seeks to condemn property, enforce building codes, or revoke a professional license. But whether a case is civil or criminal, the trial court makes the initial decisions, or "rulings." Those rulings can then be appealed to the appellate courts (Courts of appeal or Supreme Courts).

The vast majority of cases in which a Forensic Anthropologist will be involved are criminal cases, particularly for those professionals who are associated with a medical examiner or coroner's office. This correlation exists because the nature of the work – biological profile, trauma analysis, postmortem interval duration, scene recoveries and/or victim identification – is most often brought to bear on criminal investigations. However, the focus on criminal investigation does not preclude a Forensic Anthropologist's participation in civil matters (for example, a wrongful death case or mishandling of human remains by a funeral home).

## 9.2   Understanding the judicial process

The judicial system in the United States is based on an adversarial process. Simply stated, this means that two or more "sides" with an interest in the outcome will have an opportunity to present evidence in support of their position, and also to test the evidence presented by the other side(s). In theory, this manner of presentation of evidence will allow a fact finder (sometimes also called "the trier of fact"), usually a jury but sometimes a judge, to determine what the facts are. The fact finder must then apply the law to those facts in order to reach a decision (in the case of a jury, this is known as returning a verdict). In a criminal case, the "sides" will usually be a prosecutor (e.g. a county attorney, district attorney, assistant attorney general, assistant United States attorney, etc.) and a defense attorney (e.g. a public defender, legal defender, private attorney, etc.). The prosecutor's job, generally speaking, is to present evidence that demonstrates that a crime has been committed and that the defendant is responsible. The defense attorney's job, also generally speaking, is to cast doubt on the prosecutor's evidence or to present an alternative theory of the case.

In a civil case, the "sides" will usually be one or more "plaintiffs," and one or more "defendants" (or "respondents"). The plaintiff is the party bringing the claim, while the defendant is (as the name implies) the party defending against the claim. In most civil cases, a Forensic Anthropologist is involved as a retained expert for one of the "sides" because the anthropologist's opinion is believed to support that party's position in the case. Civil cases can quickly become complicated with the addition of multiple plaintiffs, multiple defendants, and multiple claims. Generally, though, practitioners need not worry about the complexities of civil practice, as the number of parties and claims in a case rarely impacts the specific work the Forensic Anthropologist is asked to perform.

The judge oversees the adversarial process in both criminal and civil cases. There are many rules that guide the judge, such as rules of procedure and rules of evidence. These rules vary from state to state, but the basic framework is very similar (particularly in the rules of evidence). There is also what is known as "substantive law." In criminal cases, "substantive law" defines the elements of the crime with which a person has been charged (and any defenses to that charge). Similarly, in civil cases, "substantive law" defines the elements of the plaintiff's claims (and also any defenses to those claims). The substantive law is found in both statutes (written laws) and written decisions published by appellate courts (including state and federal courts of appeal and supreme courts). The body of written court decisions is commonly referred to as the "common law" or "precedent."

### 9.2.1  The criminal process
*Note, the following description is simplified, and is intended only as a general overview of the criminal process. Practitioners should familiarize themselves as best as they are able with the procedures that apply in the jurisdiction in which they work. Practitioners should also be mindful that the vast majority of criminal cases are resolved prior to trial, either by plea agreement or dismissal of charges.*

### 9.2.1.1  Pretrial
The criminal process generally begins with an investigation by a police or other law enforcement agency (Figure 9.2). In the state system, the police agency is often a local agency, such as a municipal police department or a Sheriff's or Marshall's office (though there are many others). Alternatively, the agency may be a statewide office, such as a department of public safety or bureau of investigation. In the federal system, the police agency with which a Forensic Anthropologist most typically will interact is the Federal Bureau of Investigation, or perhaps Immigration and Customs Enforcement (ICE) or Border Patrol, but there are many other investigative agencies such as, for example, the Drug Enforcement Administration or Secret Service.

If the investigating agency believes there is sufficient evidence of a crime, the case will be referred to a prosecuting agency. The job of the prosecuting agency is to assess the evidence and determine whether specific criminal charges should be filed. If the prosecuting agency elects to file charges directly, it will typically do so through a charging document known as a "complaint." Alternatively, the prosecuting agency may refer the matter to a grand jury. A grand jury is a group of

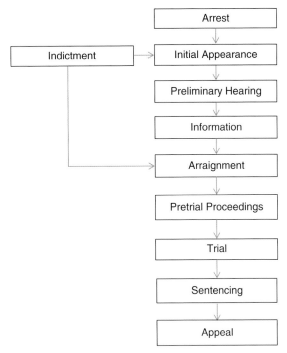

**Figure 9.2** Simplified order of proceedings in a criminal case.

citizens authorized by law to conduct investigations and return charges by way of a charging document known as an "indictment" or a "presentment." Many jurisdictions employ a dual system through which criminal charges may be brought either by complaint or indictment. See generally LaFave et al. (2017), section 13.1 (Nature of the decision whether to prosecute).

In most cases, a person accused of a crime will be placed under arrest and brought before the court. Practitioners should be aware that there can be a significant lag time between the commission of a crime, the investigation of that crime, and a subsequent arrest. A criminal suspect's first court appearance following arrest is known as an "initial appearance." The purpose of the initial appearance, generally speaking, is to advise the accused of the charge(s) against him or her, appoint counsel (if the accused cannot afford a lawyer), and determine any conditions of release. See, e.g. Federal Rules of Criminal Procedure (Fed. R. Crim. P.), Rule 5.

If the person has been accused of a felony (as will most often be the case in matters in which a Forensic Anthropologist is involved), the next step is to determine whether there is sufficient evidence to support a finding of probable cause that the accused committed the crime(s) with which he or she has been charged. This determination is most typically made at a hearing known as a "preliminary hearing." See, e.g. Fed. R. Crim. P, Rule 5.1. If probable cause is found to exist, and the case began with the filing of a complaint, the prosecuting agency will prepare and file a formal set of charges known as an "information." If the case began with an indictment, the indictment serves as the formal charging document. Whether the case proceeds by information or indictment, the next step in the process is the "arraignment," at which time formal criminal charges will be entered and the accused asked to plead to those charges. See, e.g. Fed. R. Crim. P, Rule 10. In most cases, that plea will be "not guilty."

At the conclusion of the arraignment (assuming a plea of "not guilty"), the case will be placed on the court's calendar, either for trial or a pretrial proceeding at which a trial will be set. Depending on the nature of the charges and the complexity of the case, there can be any number of pretrial proceedings. Generally, though, if a Forensic Anthropologist is involved, the case involves a death, and so by definition will be among the most serious of cases brought before the court.

The filing of the charging document triggers not only certain procedural rights for the person accused of a crime, but also a process of exchanging information known as "discovery." Think of "discovery" as the tools available to lawyers (and persons who represent themselves) to discover information about the case. One of the most common of these tools is a written request for documents, which may or may not include a subpoena. A subpoena is a court order that commands the person who receives it to produce the documents (or persons or other things) that are identified in the subpoena. Subpoenas are often necessary, but not always. The parties to a criminal prosecution frequently reach voluntary agreements for the disclosure of information that is being requested (and in many cases the prosecution has an affirmative duty to disclose such information). Parties also may conduct formal and informal interviews. The formal interview, known as a deposition, is conducted under oath in the presence of a court reporter, and results in a transcript of the deponent's sworn testimony (see Section 9.3 for further discussion of depositions).

### 9.2.1.2 Trial

The right to trial by jury in a criminal case is guaranteed by the Constitution (Amendment 6), and the vast majority of criminal trials are jury trials. Criminal trials generally proceed in the following order. First, the parties will select a jury. Jury selection proceeds through a series of questions and answers commonly known as "voir dire." The goal of jury selection is to identify any potential jurors who have knowledge about the case or any of the persons involved in it, to find out if any potential jurors have preconceived opinions about the case which they might find difficult to set aside, and to find out if any potential jurors have had any personal or family experiences that might cause them to identify with one or another of the parties. Jury selection can be a time consuming process, particularly in more serious cases such as homicides. Forensic Anthropologists who have been subpoenaed to appear early in a trial should inquire whether their presence is required on days that jury selection is taking place (the answer should be "no").

After jury selection is complete, the judge will provide the jury with preliminary instructions outlining the nature of the case and the manner in which the trial will proceed. Next, the prosecuting attorney will make an opening statement giving the jury a preview of the case. The defense counsel (or defendant, if they represent themselves) may make an opening statement outlining the defense case after the prosecutor's statement; in some jurisdictions, the defense may postpone its opening statement until after the prosecutor's case has been presented. Opening statements are not evidence, nor are they argument. The purpose of an opening statement is to help the jury prepare for anticipated evidence.

Next, the prosecution (government) will present its case through evidence consisting of witness testimony, documents, and/or tangible items (such as, for example, a weapon or clothing). After the prosecution finishes the presentation of its evidence, the defendant may present evidence. The defendant is not required to present evidence (and in many cases chooses not to), as the prosecution has the burden to prove the charges brought. If the defendant does produce evidence, the prosecution is permitted to present additional, or "rebuttal" evidence, after the defendant's case. With each witness, there are three rounds of examination: a direct examination by the side who calls the witness, a cross-examination by the opposing side, and, finally, a redirect examination. This usually ends the testimony of that witness, although the judge may allow additional examination. In some jurisdictions, the jury is allowed to submit questions as well.

After all of the evidence is presented, the judge will give the jury final instructions, including the rules of law the jury must apply to the facts in order to reach a verdict. Next, the parties will make closing arguments. The purpose of a closing argument is to review the evidence presented and the applicable law, and argue to the jury why, in the prosecutor's or defendant's view, the jury should either convict or acquit. In most (if not all) jurisdictions, the government has the right to open and close the argument because the government has the burden of proof. The standard of proof in a criminal case is very high. Jurors are instructed that the government must prove its case "beyond a reasonable doubt." Stated another way, this standard requires proof that leaves the jury firmly convinced of the defendant's guilt.

Once the closing arguments are completed, the jury will deliberate in private. In a criminal case, the verdict must be unanimous. See, e.g. Fed. R. Crim. P., Rule 31(a). If the jury reaches a unanimous verdict, the verdict is read or "returned" in open court with the parties present. Juries are usually able to reach a unanimous verdict, but that does not always happen. If the jury is unable to reach a verdict, the judge may provide additional instructions, and/or the parties may be permitted to present additional arguments. If the jury is still unable to reach a verdict, the judge will declare a mistrial for what is often called a "hung jury." In that case, it is up to the prosecutor to decide whether to seek a new trial.

If a defendant is found not guilty (acquitted), the judge will order the defendant released (assuming there are no other charges pending). If the defendant is found guilty, the defendant will be set for sentencing. At sentencing, the Court will enter a formal judgment of guilt and apply whatever sentence is prescribed for the offense for which the defendant has been convicted. The Court usually has discretion to enter a sentence within a prescribed range (such as a prison term between 5 years and 15 years). The severity (or leniency) of the sentence depends on the specific facts and circumstances of the case.

### 9.2.1.3  Appeal

A defendant who is convicted of a crime has the right to appeal. The purpose of an appeal is, at root, to ensure that the defendant received a fair trial. If the Court or the parties committed errors that violated the defendant's right to receive a fair trial, the case may be returned (remanded) to the trial court for further proceedings, up through and including a new trial. The Forensic Anthropologist will rarely participate in the appeal process, because it is based on a review of the trial record rather than new evidence. There may, however, be times when a Forensic Anthropologist is asked to consult on the trial record in order to assist counsel in preparing the appellate briefs.

Another type of "appeal" on the criminal side is a process known as post-conviction relief. In this instance, the defendant files a petition with the trial court in which he or she presents arguments as to why his or her conviction should be overturned. One of the most common arguments presented in a petition for post-conviction relief is ineffective assistance of counsel, but others include lack of jurisdiction, improper sentencing, and newly discovered evidence. Similar to a true appeal (i.e. an appeal to a court of appeals), the Forensic Anthropologist is unlikely to participate directly in a proceeding for post-conviction relief. However, the possibility for such participation exists, as the trial court may, if deemed appropriate, conduct an evidentiary hearing on a petition for post-conviction relief (Figure 9.3).

### 9.2.2  The civil process

### 9.2.2.1  Pretrial

The civil process generally begins with the filing of a civil complaint. The complaint identifies the parties to the case and the basis for the Court's jurisdiction,

Case example: PCR evidentiary hearing

A Forensic Anthropologist was contacted by the
Prosecutor who was defending a PCR
request from an inmate based on evidence recovered
during the investigation. The Forensic Anthropologist
had been involved in a body recovery from a desert
location. The body had been hidden under a large
electrical wire spool; dry lye was used to disguise the
smell. The area of recovery was covered with
ammunition from private gun owners. During the course
of the recovery a projectile was inadvertently included
in the body pouch with the decedent. The defendant
argued that the second projectile had not been tested and
implicated a second shooter. The Forensic
Anthropologist was called to testify about the process of
recovery and the autopsy proceedings as well as to
testify about the condition of the projectile. PCR was
denied by the Judge.

**Figure 9.3**  Post-conviction relief (PCR) evidentiary hearing expert testimony example.

and should contain a short and plain statement of the grounds for the complaint (i.e. the nature of the dispute between the parties) and the relief that is being requested. Once a copy of the complaint has been provided to ("served on") the defendant, the defendant is required to file a responsive pleading called an answer. The answer serves to admit or deny the allegations in the complaint, and raise defenses to each claim that is asserted. Sometimes a defendant will file some other response to a complaint (such as a motion to dismiss); however, the manner in which the early stages of the case are defined will rarely impact the work that a Forensic Anthropologist conducts in a civil matter.

After the complaint and answer are filed (there may be other pleadings such as counterclaims or third party complaints, but the complaint and answer form the basic structure), the parties engage in "discovery" similar to that conducted in a criminal case (see above). In civil cases, discovery may include written questions ("interrogatories"), or requests that the opposing party make certain admissions. See, e.g. Federal Rules of Civil Procedure (Fed. R. Civ. P.), Rules 33 and 36. Discovery in civil cases can often be extensive, and as to a Forensic Anthropologist retained as an expert, will likely involve, at minimum, requests for documents and formal deposition testimony (see below).

After the parties have gathered information about the case, any number of pretrial motions may be filed. One of the most common is the motion for summary judgment. See, e.g. Fed R. Civ. P. 56. A motion for summary judgment argues to the Court that there are no genuine issues of material fact in the case, and that the moving party is entitled to judgment as a matter of law. Motions for summary judgment often implicate expert testimony, because that testimony (usually in the form of a sworn affidavit or declaration) can be used to bolster the moving party's position. Contrariwise, such testimony also can be used to show that summary judgment is not appropriate because there are genuine issues of material fact present in the case.

Over the life of a civil case, the judge will make various rulings that define the issues that must be set for trial. Once the point is reached where the key issues are defined, the judge will confer with the parties, find out how long the trial is expected to last, and set the case for trial. As is the case with criminal matters, civil suits are usually tried to a jury. However, the parties may (and sometimes must) choose to have a "bench" trial, in which the case is tried to the judge instead of a jury.

### 9.2.2.2 Trial

Similar to criminal cases, parties to a civil matter are entitled to a trial by jury, and demands for jury trials are made as a matter of routine upon the filing of a complaint. As is the case with criminal trials, the parties will select a jury, the judge will provide the jury with preliminary instructions, the parties will make opening statements, the plaintiff will present evidence, the defendant will present evidence, the judge will give final instructions, the parties will make closing arguments, and the jury will deliberate and return a verdict. Unlike criminal cases, the jury's verdict in a civil case need not be unanimous. The general rule is a three-fourths majority (note, however, that in federal court, all verdicts, whether civil or criminal, must be unanimous. See, e.g. Fed. R. Civ. P., Rule 48(b) and Fed. R. Crim. P., Rule 31(a)). After the jury returns its verdict, and the parties have had an opportunity to be heard, the judge will enter a final judgment. That final judgment may then be appealed.

Civil cases are subject to a lower standard of proof. Whereas in criminal cases the standard is proof beyond a reasonable doubt, the standard in civil cases is preponderance of the evidence ("more probably true than not true"). Some claims are subject to a higher standard known as clear and convincing evidence ("highly probable"), but that standard still is not as high as the criminal standard.

### 9.2.2.3 Appeal

Like criminal cases, an appeal in a civil matter looks to the fairness of the trial (or the judge's decisions in the case, if final rulings are made short of trial). Typically, however, an appeal in a civil matter focuses on discrete legal issues and whether the trial court properly applied the law. Similar to criminal matters, if the appeal is upheld, the case may be returned to the trial court for further proceedings, up through and including a new trial.

## 9.3   The role of the forensic anthropologist

### 9.3.1   Criminal cases

A Forensic Anthropologist's role in a criminal case usually will begin in the investigatory phase, i.e. well in advance of the referral to the prosecuting agency and the filing of charges. For that reason, the Forensic Anthropologist may not necessarily be thinking of the legal ramifications of his or her work. However, the best practice is to approach each case with a view toward the end result: a trial before a jury. The practitioner should assume that all of his or her analysis and written work product will be subjected to rigorous review and scrutiny, including review and scrutiny by another Forensic Anthropologist.

Most Forensic Anthropologists who consult on cases that may result in criminal charges prepare a written report of their findings and conclusions (see Chapter 6). The importance of proper report writing cannot be overstated, because the report sets the stage for all of the Forensic Anthropologist's subsequent testimony. A good rule of thumb is that reports should be written with the expectation that they will end up in front of a jury. Applying that rule, it follows that reports should be concise, well-organized, and spell-checked. A badly written report reflects poorly on the author's credibility, and credibility is an issue that can be raised (and often is) at many points during the life of a case. As the case progresses, the anthropologist may be asked to amend his or her report to reflect additional evidence that has been uncovered. The best practice in this situation is to write a supplemental report, and explain in that supplemental report the reason it is being prepared. The existence of supplemental reports is not a bad thing, but the practitioner should always be able to explain why he or she prepared one.

As set forth above, there are several methods by which criminal charges may be brought. In the case of a direct complaint (or similar charging document), the prosecutor's office may consider the Forensic Anthropologist's report and/or consult with the Forensic Anthropologist in advance of filing charges. In the event of a grand jury investigation or a coroner's inquest (a cause of death determination conducted by a coroner), the Forensic Anthropologist could be called directly as a testifying witness (though this is unlikely). At these early stages, the role of the anthropologist is fairly limited – essentially testifying to the contents of his or her report in order to establish a factual basis for whatever charges might be filed.

If criminal charges are filed, the Forensic Anthropologist who worked on the case will be disclosed to the defense as a potential witness, or at least as a person with relevant knowledge. Similarly, the Forensic Anthropologist's report and any other formal work product also will be disclosed. There is an important observation to be made here: the Forensic Anthropologist initially involved in the case is most typically listed as a prosecution witness because the prosecutor has determined, at least in part on the Forensic Anthropologist's report, that grounds exist to support criminal charges. But, the fact that one side or another identifies the anthropologist as a potential witness does not change the fundamental role of the anthropologist, which, as a scientific expert, is to remain neutral and to convey information in a professional and objective manner. There is often a temptation to choose a "right" side, but that temptation must always be avoided. Not only does such conduct cloud objectivity, it almost always diminishes credibility. "Generally speaking, a witness has no business to concern himself with the merits of the case in which he is called on to give evidence or whether, when given, it will be material to the cause" (*Langley v. Fisher* 1843).

In some cases, the findings of the Forensic Anthropologist are a better fit for the defense theory of the case. In those situations, the roles are reversed and the prosecution will conduct pretrial interviews and cross-examination at trial. Regardless of whether the defense or the prosecution calls the expert, the imperative is to remain objective, calm, and factual in order to provide reliable information to the finders of fact. Following disclosure, the defense may choose to interview the anthropologist. Such interviews may be (and often are) relatively informal in nature, with little more than a digital recorder on the table. However, the defense also may choose to conduct a more formal interview under oath and in the presence of a court reporter. These more formal interviews are often referred to as "depositions," and because they are taken under oath, the anthropologist's answers constitute sworn testimony that may be used in later proceedings. For this reason, the anthropologist must carefully prepare for any interview, but particularly sworn testimony, by thoroughly reviewing in advance all of the particulars of the case. As a general rule, the prosecutor will want to be present during any interview, formal or not. At the conclusion of the deposition, the court reporter will prepare a written transcript of the testimony. The witness has the right to review the transcript for errors and to make changes. Do not pass up this opportunity. While review can be time consuming, court reporters are human and make mistakes, and the transcript should be accurate. There is typically a deadline associated with the submission of corrections and the anthropologist must adhere to it. This step is critical in the process.

Once the defense has had an opportunity to assess the Forensic Anthropologist's findings, the defense may choose to retain their own expert by engaging another Forensic Anthropologist. In this event, the same rules apply: if the anthropologist is listed as a defense witness, the prosecutor is able to access the anthropologist's report, and may conduct an informal or formal interview with the anthropologist. The same professional rules apply as well, i.e. the anthropologist is not an advocate; instead, his or her role is to independently assess the evidence and render objective findings based on that evidence in order to ensure that the defendant receives a fair trial. The potential presence of a second expert in any given case reinforces the importance of a thorough initial investigation and carefully prepared report and findings (see Chapter 11).

Prior to trial, either side may choose to challenge the Forensic Anthropologist's credentials and findings under the rules of evidence through what is known colloquially as a *Frye* or *Daubert* hearing (see Chapter 1). If a Frye or *Daubert* challenge is made, the goal of that challenge is to limit, or exclude in its entirety, the Forensic Anthropologist's testimony. A *Frye* or *Daubert* hearing may cover multiple points, but as a general rule the issues presented will be (i) whether the Forensic Anthropologist qualifies as an expert "by knowledge, skill, experience, training, or education," (ii) whether the Forensic Anthropologist's "scientific, technical, or other specialized knowledge" will help the jury (or the judge) understand the evidence or determine a fact in issue, and (iii) whether the techniques employed by the Forensic Anthropologist are generally accepted as reliable in the scientific community. In *Daubert* jurisdictions, the inquiry extends to (i) whether the testimony is based on sufficient facts or data, (ii) whether the testimony is the product of reliable principles and methods, and (iii) whether the Forensic Anthropologist has reliably applied the principles and methods to the facts of the case. See generally Federal Rules of Evidence (Fed. R. Evid.), Rule 702.

*Frye* and *Daubert* hearings are serious matters, and require careful preparation. When one's credentials and work product come under close scrutiny, particularly when the expert knows that the grounds for the challenge come from a professional colleague guiding the opposing counsel, there is a strong temptation to view the critique as a personal attack. As the justice system is, for better or for worse, adversarial in nature, strong policy reasons exist for ensuring that evidence presented to a jury is reliable. This element of reliability is that with which the judge will be most concerned. The practitioner should bear in mind that from the Court's perspective, the adversarial system is most effective when each side is permitted to present evidence in support of their position, and that preclusion of evidence is the exception rather than the rule. That said, the possibility of a *Frye* or *Daubert* hearing in any given case should serve as a reminder of the need for scientific rigor and integrity in each and every case on which the Forensic Anthropologist works.

While *Frye* and *Daubert* hearings are the most significant pretrial hearings in which the Forensic Anthropologist may participate, practitioners should be aware that there are other types of hearings in which their testimony may be required prior to trial. Capital (death penalty) cases present a particular area of law in which a Forensic Anthropologist may be called to testify on pretrial matters. For example, a Forensic Anthropologist might be called to provide fact testimony on whether probable cause exists to support the aggravating factors alleged in support of imposing the death penalty. Regardless of the type of hearing, however, it is important to remember that in any court hearing at which testimony is taken, such testimony may later be used at trial to support or contradict ("impeach") the anthropologist's trial testimony.

If a criminal case does not resolve by plea agreement and/or dismissal of charges, the trial is set. The side that listed the Forensic Anthropologist as a witness should provide ample advance notice of the trial dates to avoid potential conflicts. In some jurisdictions, trial subpoenas issue as a matter of course, but they should reflect dates and times previously discussed. Often, the subpoena will list the start date of the trial instead of the date of the anthropologist's intended testimony. The anthropologist should seek clarification of the actual date and time they are needed. Courts and counsel should be sensitive to professional schedules, but this does not always occur; therefore, clear communication is key.

On the date set for testimony, the Forensic Anthropologist should arrive reasonably early to address any last minute matters that may have arisen, and to gather their thoughts. While discussed in more detail below in Section 9.4, the importance of professional dress cannot be overstated – there is no second chance to make a first impression. Court rules may require witnesses to wait outside the courtroom before giving testimony (often referred to as the "rule of exclusion"), although experts sometimes are permitted to be present inside the courtroom. The attorney that called the anthropologist should explain this process in advance of trial. The anthropologist should also be aware that this waiting period is not fixed and there are many circumstances where the waiting period is lengthy. Indeed, the anthropologist may not be called to the stand at all on the day appointed so being prepared to stay more than one day is essential. Such delays may be due to prolonged questioning of a prior witness or various motions that need to be resolved prior to the expert's appearance.

Once the Court is ready, the attorney will "call" the witness to the stand, and the witness will be sworn in front of the Clerk (Figure 9.4). The swearing in requires the witness to raise his or her right hand, and answer "yes" to some version of the following oath: "Do you solemnly swear or affirm that you will tell the truth, the whole truth, and nothing but the truth?" See, e.g. Fed. R. Evid., Rule 603 (witness must "give an oath or affirmation to testify truthfully," and oath "must be in a form designed to impress that duty on the witness's conscience"). After being sworn, the witness will be directed to take a seat in the witness box. The anthropologist should take a few moments at this time to ensure he or she is comfortable and ready to proceed. If reading glasses are necessary, be sure to bring them! Any items brought into the courtroom are subject to inspection by the opposing side, so experts are encouraged not to bring anything extraneous

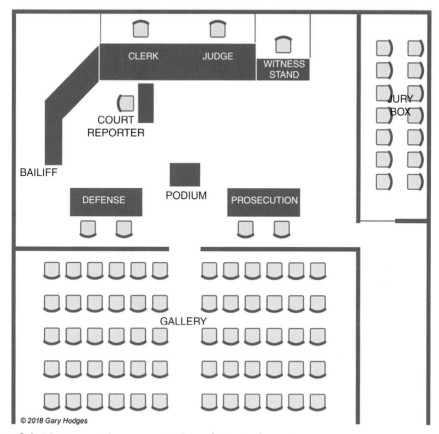

© 2018 Gary Hodges

**Figure 9.4** Diagrammatic representation of a typical courtroom.

into the courtroom. The best practice is to leave personal case files and notes, purses/bags, and any electronics (including cell phones) outside the courtroom, with the counsel's investigator, or in the car to avoid complications in the testimony. It is also possible to make a separate copy of the report, curriculum vitae, and any important material if those are needed to refresh one's memory on the witness stand.

### 9.3.1.1   Direct examination

As set forth above in the general description of criminal trial procedure, the first phase of examination is the direct examination. "Direct," as it is informally called, allows the attorney to walk the expert through the work that was completed on the case and the report that summarizes the expert's findings. Questions on direct should be, as the name implies, succinct and open-ended. Direct examination is often the practitioner's first introduction to the jury and the judge, so the opening questions usually focus on the expert's education and training (the issue of whether the practitioner qualifies as an expert generally will have been decided before trial, so the background simply lays a foundation for the expert's opinions). As trial testimony can be stressful (nervousness is normal), the initial line of questions is also an opportunity to become more comfortable with testifying, and to connect with the jury. Standard questions might address education, employment, whether the witness holds any professional licenses or certifications (board or otherwise), publications and any other professional accomplishments, and whether the witness has previously testified in court. Commonly, one of the initial questions after the vetting of credentials is "what is Forensic Anthropology and how does it apply in this case"? A succinct, easy to understand answer should be prepared in advance. Likewise, the anthropologist should be able to summarize the specific work on the case in a few sentences using lay language for the jury.

The most important rule of direct examination (and in fact any testimony) is to carefully listen to the question that is asked, and answer only that question. Witnesses are often tempted to expand or elaborate on their own, or answer the question they think the attorney is asking. This practice, however, must be avoided for two important reasons. First, the judge may have set limits on the specific types of testimony and other evidence that are permissible in the trial. If this occurs (and it is common), the attorney should already have reviewed those rulings with the expert, but testimony beyond the scope of the question asked may nonetheless run afoul of those rulings and could, in extreme cases, result in a mistrial. Secondly, if an expert expands, on his or own initiative, the scope of their testimony, they may inadvertently open avenues of cross-examination for which they (or the attorney who called them) are not properly prepared.

The second most important rule of direct examination (and a corollary to the first) is if a question is confusing, do not be embarrassed to ask for clarification. Recall that the first duty of an expert witness is to allow the fact finder to understand the basis for the expert's findings and conclusions. Matters that are common to the expert in day to day practice may be wholly foreign to the persons sitting in the courtroom, and questions designed to elucidate those matters may not always be artfully crafted. Therefore, if there is any doubt as to what is being asked, the expert should feel free to ask the attorney to clarify, repeat, or rephrase.

During the course of examination, the attorneys will more than likely ask multiple questions about the expert's report. As a general matter, court rules do not permit an expert to answer questions directly from his or her report, therefore, the best practice is to carefully review the report (and any other relevant materials) prior to providing testimony. If necessary, an expert may refresh his or her recollection during testimony by requesting to review the report that was submitted as an exhibit (see below on exhibits). There is nothing wrong with doing so, but again, in keeping with the rule, the witness will need to testify from his or her refreshed recollection rather than reading directly from the report. Practices vary significantly between jurisdictions, and some courts enforce the refreshed recollection rule more strictly than others. The expert should check with the attorney prior to testimony to determine how much they will be able to rely on looking at their report while on the stand. In general, witnesses are not permitted to act until given permission by the Judge. This prohibition includes viewing photographs, marking photographs (if projected), standing to illustrate a point or looking at their report. The expert may ask the attorney if the report can be viewed to refresh memory, allowing the attorney to ask permission from the judge. The rule here, however, is to wait for the answer before opening the report or other items.

In most criminal cases in which a Forensic Anthropologist is involved, there are likely to be a number of exhibits. The term "exhibits" refers to documents, photographs, and other things that are offered into evidence. Each exhibit is "marked" – identified by a number or letter – to ensure a clear record of the proceedings. The lawyers may agree to the admission of exhibits, but not always. In that event, the lawyer seeking to admit the exhibit must elicit testimony that the exhibit is what it purports to be, and demonstrate its relevance to the proceedings. In the context of forensic testimony, the anthropologist may be asked to identify his or her report, and any number of supporting documents (notes, photographs, radiographs, etc.) prior to those items being admitted into evidence. On those occasions, the anthropologist should review each exhibit to ensure its completeness and accuracy. When examining photographs that have not yet been admitted, the witness should take great care to prevent jurors from viewing them. The judge is the final arbiter of whether evidence is admissible or not. In a jury trial, the jury is not allowed to consider evidence that has not been admitted into the record.

Similarly, in cases where the defendant is being tried a second time due to a mistrial, hung jury or additional charges, the previous testimony is sacrosanct; that is, the expert may not refer to the trial or their role in it. Doing so may result in a mistrial (Figure 9.5). Typically counsel will alert the expert prior to going into the courtroom but not always. In some instances, the language from a deposition or pretrial interview will be lumped in with the previous trial testimony and all referred to as "previous testimony." The jury will not decipher that a trial occurred when this technique is employed. The rule of thumb is to govern words when speaking.

### 9.3.1.2  Cross-examination

Following the completion of direct examination, the opposing attorney will have the opportunity for cross-examination ("cross" for short). Cross-examination is

Retrial in capital murder case

Q: When you examined the skeletal remains did you find any trauma to the bones?

A: Yes, as you recall I testified previously that I found sharp force defects in the body of the second cervical vertebra and in the facial skeleton.

DC: Judge, may we approach.

Judge: Yes.

DC: I am requesting a mistrial due to the fact that this witness revealed that there was a previous trial.

PA: Judge, the slip was minimal and could have been referring to the pretrial interview, therefore a mistrial is not warranted.

Judge: OK, I will table the request for now until we see how the rest of the testimony transpires.

ASIDE TO WITNESS: Remember you are precluded from referring to any previous trials in this case.

**Figure 9.5** Example of trial testimony with potential for mistrial.

very different from direct examination. For one thing, an attorney on cross is able to, and often exclusively will, ask leading questions. Think of a leading question as a question that also contains the answer – the witness is asked only to answer "yes" or "no," or "correct" or "incorrect," without being able to elaborate further. Through the use of leading questions, an attorney on cross-examination will endeavor to very carefully guide and control the witness's testimony.

Cross-examination can be a very frustrating experience, as the witness is typically incapable of providing context to the "yes" or "no" answers that are given. However, practitioners should resist the urge to argue. If a yes or no answer is not possible, then say so. If a question is confusing, say so and ask that it be clarified or rephrased. Above all, stay calm and remember to listen carefully to each question asked. Keep in mind that at the conclusion of cross-examination, there will be an opportunity to provide further explanation on redirect examination (see Section 9.3.1.3), and clean up any potential misimpressions.

Often, one of the goals on cross-examination is to reduce the credibility of a witness in the eyes of the jury or the judge. This tactic is an outgrowth of the adversarial process, and seeks to diminish the weight of the witness's testimony so as to increase the weight of any opposing testimony. Attacks on credibility often begin with the witness's credentials. Questions in this vein might include whether the witness has had any academic or professional discipline, whether they have had any license or certification revoked or suspended, or whether they ever have been the subject of any ethical complaints or proceedings. Usually, there is an explanation for these types of issues, and the best practice is to bring them out in the friendlier environment of direct examination so as not to leave the impression with the jury that the expert has something to hide. The last place any witness wants something like this to come out for the first time is in trial. If there's an issue, make sure it is disclosed early. One of the more common strategies employed is addressing a PhD-holding Forensic Anthropologist as Mr., Mrs., Miss or Ms. Likewise many attorneys will ask the question, "you are not a medical doctor, correct?" The best response is to merely acknowledge that fact. Some practitioners will correct an attorney who does not address them according to convention, but this can have the opposite of the desired effect and reduce the credibility of the witness in the eyes of the jury. Finally, an attorney on cross-examination may ask whether the expert has testified more for the defense or the prosecution in other cases, in an effort to suggest that the expert tends to favor one side over another. Answers to these questions should be direct and truthful; it may be useful to have some basic statistics at hand.

A second line of attack on an expert's credibility goes to the underlying examination and accompanying report. Any potential errors or deficiencies – real or creatively imagined – will be raised. The anthropologist may be questioned about alternative methodologies or interpretations, or presented with academic treatises and asked why he or she did not rely on them. The anthropologist may be asked how many cases they have examined, how many of this type of case or how many of this type of trauma. Having those numbers in mind is helpful. Often, the anthropologist will be presented with the findings and/or critiques of the opposing expert, the suggestion being that the approach employed was incorrect or substandard. There are any number of avenues by which the practitioner's professional opinions will be tested. Again, this is part and parcel of the adversarial system, and should be recognized as such. The key is to maintain a calm demeanor, acknowledge errors if they exist (jurors are human and do not expect perfection), and acknowledge, when appropriate, alternative approaches or outcomes.

One particularly effective method of cross-examination involves impeachment with prior inconsistent statements. In this scenario, if a witness makes a statement at trial that is inconsistent with prior testimony (such as, for example, during a deposition or in an affidavit), the rules of evidence allow the attorney on cross to bring that inconsistency to the attention of the jury. The impact of prior inconsistent statements on a witness's credibility can be significant, and underscores the need to testify consistently based on the available scientific evidence and to review any existing interview transcripts or affidavit statements prior to testifying.

### 9.3.1.3  Redirect examination

Once cross-examination is concluded, the attorney who first called the witness will have the opportunity to ask additional questions. This last line of examination is known as redirect. The primary purpose of redirect is to allow the witness to clarify or elaborate on testimony provided during cross-examination. In keeping with this purpose, court rules typically limit the attorney's questions only to those matters that were raised on cross; redirect is not an opportunity to explore new themes or evidence. The witness should bear this in mind when answering any questions during this phase. Generally speaking, redirect examination is the last phase of testimony, after which the witness is excused. In certain cases, the judge may allow "re-cross" and additional redirect, but this is uncommon.

### 9.3.1.4  Jury and judge questions

In some jurisdictions, the jury is allowed to ask questions of witnesses, and rarely, the Judge may ask a question. Local practices vary, but as a general rule, in those jurisdictions that allow jury questions, the questions are asked after the completion of redirect examination. The judge will first screen the questions to ensure they comply with the rules of evidence, and allow the lawyers an opportunity to object. If the question is permissible, it will be asked of the witness. Usually, the lawyers will be allowed to ask follow-up questions. Juror questions are often very perceptive, touching on matters the lawyers may have missed or even tried to avoid. Jury questions also provide good "teaching moments," and the Forensic Anthropologist should not shy away from taking advantage of those moments. Attorneys are chary of precluding juror questions and in many cases the queries cut to the heart of the matter and make it easier for the expert to overcome a frustrating cross-examination.

### 9.3.2  Civil cases

Civil cases come in all shapes and sizes, but the universe of civil cases in which a Forensic Anthropologist is likely to be involved is quite small. More likely than not, the case will be one for wrongful death, where the anthropologist's testimony bears on identification, trauma analysis, and/or postmortem interval. Other possible types of cases include human factors in motor vehicle or pedestrian fatalities, types of bone trauma observed in living children, or age-at-death estimations in police custody or border patrol cases as the outcome differs if the individual is over 18 years of age. Claims may also be made regarding handling of a body by a funeral home or commingling of cremated remains.

The Forensic Anthropologist's role in a civil case is very similar to that of a criminal case to the extent that the anthropologist provides specific expertise that helps explain the relevant facts, and helps the lawyers understand and assess the relative strengths and weaknesses of the case. However, the posture of a civil case is different in that the anthropologist is being retained by one side or the other with a specific view toward supporting that party's theory of the case. This posture can at times lead to conflict, as attorneys will, as a general rule, endeavor to frame the scientific testimony in a way that most benefits their client. This process of framing the case may place the anthropologist in a position in which he or she is asked to opine on matters beyond the scope of his or her practice, or beyond the reasonable limits of the scientific evidence. Thus, clarity at the outset is critical.

If a Forensic Anthropologist is asked to work on a civil case, one of the first questions that should be asked is the scope of the engagement. Generally speaking, the engagement will be either as a consulting expert or a testifying expert. A consulting expert is (as the name implies) not expected to testify; rather, his or her role is to help the attorneys understand the evidence in the case. This role will typically include a review of the available evidence and any relevant literature. If the other side has retained an expert, the consulting expert almost certainly will be asked to review and comment on that expert's report (and perhaps his or her qualifications). Finally, a consulting expert may be asked to assist the lawyers at trial and provide insight into the evidence presented. Practitioners should note that during the course of their preparation for trial, attorneys may seek to convert a consulting expert to a testifying expert. All of these matters should be clarified before the work is accepted, and should be reduced to writing if possible.

The role of a testifying expert is significantly greater than that of a consulting expert inasmuch as the testifying expert performs all of the functions of the consulting expert in addition to providing testimony both before and at trial. Further, the testifying expert is retained with the express purpose of eliciting opinions that support that side's position. Thus, more often than not, the testifying expert will be asked to explicitly criticize, or at least critique, the opinions of the other side's expert. And in turn, the testifying expert and his or her work product will be the subject of close scrutiny and/or criticism from the other side's expert (see Section 9.3.1.2). The practical lesson to be drawn is that accepting this type of engagement is not a decision that should be taken lightly, as it sets the practitioner down a road that can be both long and difficult.

If a Forensic Anthropologist is asked to serve as a testifying expert, he or she should first confirm the subjects about which he or she will be asked to testify, and then ask him or herself whether those matters fairly fall within his or her expertise. The importance of self-review at the outset of any engagement cannot be overstated, as the opposing party will conduct its own investigation, and identify any areas of testimony that aren't supported by the expert's education or experience (and then bring that out at trial). If the engagement is accepted, the terms of that engagement, including the scope of expected testimony, should be obtained in writing.

As a general rule, testifying experts are required to produce reports, which then must be disclosed to the opposing side. Accordingly, the Forensic Anthropologist should apply equal rigor to the preparation of his or her report in a civil matter, as it will be the subject of close scrutiny. In addition to written reports, testifying experts often are asked to provide sworn affidavits. Affidavits are used in a number of contexts, but in a civil case, the affidavit is most typically used to support a motion that is filed with the Court. The common practice is for the attorney to draft the affidavit, and to craft it in such a way as to best support the client's position. There is nothing inherently wrong with this practice, but it represents a potential pitfall for the expert. Once signed by the expert, the affidavit is considered to be sworn testimony by that expert, and can later be used against them. The best practice is for the Forensic Anthropologist to very carefully review any affidavit that is presented to him or her for signature, and ensure that it accurately reflects the anthropologist's findings and opinions. Sometimes an entire line of questioning can result from a single inartful turn of phrase.

Trial testimony in a civil case proceeds in a manner similar to a criminal case, with direct examination, cross-examination, redirect examination, and in some jurisdictions, jury or Judge questions (see above). Expert witnesses in a civil case also are subject to the same potential *Frye* and *Daubert* challenges as those in a criminal matter. Therefore, objective analysis and scientific rigor are paramount.

## 9.4 The courtroom: etiquette and pitfalls

Not all experts are created equal. The ability to convey complex information in a manner that is understandable by judges and jurors comes more naturally to some than others, just as some experts are more comfortable than others with the pressure of the courtroom environment (not to mention the justice system as a whole). However, experience counts, and persons who appear as witnesses on a regular or semi-regular basis will quickly find themselves better able to navigate the system and focus on their role as educators. For those with less (or no) experience, the following section provides guidance for court appearances and identifies a number of common pitfalls to avoid (Figure 9.6).

The first rule of successfully appearing in court is to project credibility. A Forensic Anthropologist testifying as an expert should always dress for court, meaning a suit or something equally formal. Some testimony will occur in more

Etiquette for Court

(1) Dress appropriately

(2) Be prepared

(3) Use plain English

(4) Use common analogies

(5) Be respectful of all parties

(6) Know and follow the rules

**Figure 9.6** Courtroom etiquette.

rural areas where formal or "fancy" dress may be off-putting or give the impression that the testimony has been bought. In these instances, quiet, appropriate clothing is recommended. In all instances jewelry for men and women should be subdued and restrained, hair should be contained and make-up should be understated. The science is the center here, not the outlandish dress of the expert. Remember – there will be no second chance to make a first impression, and first impressions count! During testimony, the anthropologist should connect with the jury by making eye contact and speaking directly to the jury when answering questions. Experience shows that some of the most effective experts will look at the attorneys while questions are being asked, and then turn to the jury to answer. Building a rapport with the jury often builds credibility. Bear in mind, however, that credibility does not just come from the witness stand. The jury (and the judge) will be observing the expert at all times while he or she is in the courtroom, and experts should conduct themselves accordingly.

All witnesses, but particularly experts, should speak clearly and concisely, and use plain English as often as possible. Technical jargon usually serves only to confuse and this includes the correct names for bones. Use of terms such as "thigh bone" or "collarbone" conveys the same information but in a language that the jurors will understand whereas "femur" and "clavicle" may communicate nothing. Refrain from using filler words such as "um" or "like"; if necessary practice standard answers to get used to speaking comfortably without pauses. Try to remain as relaxed as possible without slumping in the witness box. Convey to the jury that the facts are fully understood. Use common analogies when possible to explain more complex processes, such as using the image of an inflated balloon being impacted by a fist to explain the forces in focal blunt impact to the cranium. And, while it is permissible to insert a little humor into the testimony, tread lightly. Many verbal analogies in Forensic Pathology and Anthropology revolve around food, such as "consistency of baby food," and while this is "normal" to practitioners, others may not be amused. A trial is, after all, a serious matter with someone's freedom or even life at stake, and while being perceived as "human" is positive, being taken seriously is a necessity. The family of the victim is often present in the courtroom so questionable comments about the deceased will inflict additional pain to them. To this point many experts will humanize the victim by referring to them by name, rather than saying decedent, or body, or remains.

The second rule of successfully appearing in court is to properly prepare. While it perhaps goes without saying, preparation is key to successful testimony. If a Forensic Anthropologist is retained as an expert, he or she should review as much material in the case as possible, and fully familiarize him or herself with the evidence in the case. The practitioner should have a good working knowledge of the authorities on which he or she relies, and perhaps even more importantly, the authorities that may be used against him or her. An expert witness should recognize the strengths and weaknesses of the positions he or she has taken, and be prepared to respond to questions as to both. Prior to trial, the Forensic Anthropologist should always re-review his or her report and, as needed, the reports of other experts in the case so he or she can speak to those matters from memory where possible. Review of any relevant literature that has been published since the report was written that may be used by others is useful.

The third rule of successfully appearing in court is observing proper courtroom etiquette. Participants in court proceedings should always be respectful – respectful to the parties, the Court, the jury, the other experts, and even the attorneys (though that may be hard at times). Some common rules of thumb include (i) do not enter the courtroom until asked to do so, (ii) enter and leave the courtroom quietly, (iii) follow the judge's directions, and refer to the judge as "your honor" or "judge," (iv) be respectful to court staff, (v) do not discuss testimony with anyone other than the retaining attorney, unless asked or directed to do so, (vi) let the attorney know if demonstrative exhibits, such as models, charts, or graphs are to be used, (vii) do not refer to the report or any other written materials during testimony unless directed to do so, and (viii) if asked by the attorney to stand as part of the demonstration, be sure to have the judge's permission first.

The last rule, but certainly not the least, is that the expert should testify within the bounds of their expert knowledge. While many Forensic Anthropologists have greater than average understanding of human biology and pathology as well as mechanisms of soft tissue injury, those areas are outside the purview of their knowledge and expertise. If asked about cause of death or the hemorrhage in the soft tissue or pain associated with an injury, the Forensic Anthropologist should defer to the forensic pathologist. Allowing an attorney to "wander into the weeds" during an interview or in trial opens a trapdoor into which, unfortunately, many practitioners unwittingly stumble, sometimes with negative and long-lasting effects.

The above rules may not substitute for practical experience, but should enable the practitioner to avoid some of the more common pitfalls of court appearances, and allow for effective expert testimony.

## References

LaFave, W., Israel, J., King, N., and Kerr, O. (2017). *Criminal Procedure*, 4ee. St. Paul: West Publishing.

*Langley v. Fisher*, 5 Beav. 447 (1843).

## CHAPTER 10

# Litigation graphics in the courtroom presentation of forensic anthropology

Gary Hodges

*Maricopa County Attorney Office, Phoenix, AZ, USA*

A jury can – and perhaps *should* – be regarded as the toughest of crowds. In the professional bubbles of those who work in the criminal justice system or testify in court, it is easy to lose sight of the fact that the jury does not approach cases with the same knowledge or interest attorneys or expert witnesses do. Bubble-dwellers forget that jurors are often unhappy that this new civic responsibility is interfering with other professional, academic, caregiver, or recreational commitments. The trial's schedule might be earlier or later than they are normally out, and thus they might be half asleep. The court complex could be far out of their way and they are experiencing the baptism by fire of navigating downtown rush hour traffic for the first time, or maybe they are having to unravel a new public transit route.

Jurors are possibly more skeptical of authority, education, or expertise than ever before. A juror could have virtually any level of scientific, medical, or anatomical literacy (therefore one should play it safe and assume "none"). Our smartphone-equipped, always connected lifestyle might be leaving our typical juror feeling a little bit of withdrawal (Dscout 2016), and their expectations of evidence and testimony have been heavily influenced by the ubiquitous *Crime Scene Investigation* (CSI)-style shows and courtroom dramas that advertise astounding technology, dramatic reveals, and unambiguous evidence that makes the rest of the trial a mere formality (Schweitzer and Saks 2007). In almost every possible way, this audience – the jury – is arguably the least receptive, engaged, and amenable it could be, and is now waiting to be impressed.

Realistically, the burden of overcoming these hurdles mostly falls to the attorneys, and in particular their preparation, oratory, and the overall strength of their case. Preparation is critically important for expert witnesses as well, and the two together can negate much or all of the underlying resistance offered by a jury. But

*Forensic Anthropology and the United States Judicial System*, First Edition.
Edited by Laura C. Fulginiti, Kristen Hartnett-McCann, and Alison Galloway.
© 2019 John Wiley & Sons Ltd. Published 2019 by John Wiley & Sons Ltd.

no matter how expertly an expert witness' testimony is delivered, how powerful the evidence, or how persuasive the legal argument, verbal testimony and presentations have inherent drawbacks. Depending on the case, presenting solely orally could weaken the impact, comprehension (Shabiralyani et al. 2015) and retention of critical facts (Bigelow and Poremba 2014). Very often, the *most* critical facts, such as those presented with technical or scientific testimony, may also be the most difficult to explain clearly.

Educators have long recognized that people learn and process new information best when using a combination of their senses – not just hearing alone. And the fastest and most effective way to communicate information to human beings is visually. Our eyes are our primary approach to understanding the world around us, and an almost direct path to our minds. Information presented visually is better understood and retained than information presented orally, not to mention more persuasive: one study demonstrated that when the same presentation was delivered by the same person with and without visual aids, the one with visuals was 43% more effective at getting audience members to take action (in that case, spend their own money – the gold standard for measuring persuasion) (Vogel et al. 1986).

But while research supports this claim, the merits of visual learning are something we know intuitively from everyday experience. Presentations at work are more engaging if they have images. Text is more easily understood with diagrams and figures. Damage to your spouse's car after a fender bender is more quickly ascertained from a photo than a verbal description. The directory in a mall is another type of optimal visual aid; imagine being confronted with a series of go left-right-or-straight-from-here directions to the food court instead of a map. The power of visuals is self-evident.

While not everyone is a trained graphic designer, most people are able to appreciate and respond to the quality of an image. Even laypersons can do a fair job at saying what colors are best for, say, food packaging or the logo of a new medical clinic or a nursery – yet we often fail to consider this inherent sensitivity to basic design principles like color, composition, layout, and font are not limited to shopping or decorating – they are just as active and powerful in the mind of a juror receiving information and evaluating evidence.

Given all these well-studied and accepted points, one would expect there to be a litigation graphics specialist on staff at every major district attorney's and public defender's office, discussing presentation strategies with attorneys and helping them create polished, professional, informative, and persuasive visual aids for use in every big trial – or at the very least, giving the PowerPoint they intend to use in their closing argument a quick once-over and spit polish. Unfortunately, that is not actually the case. Only a few offices are like the Maricopa County Attorney's Office, which has two full-time litigation graphics specialists on staff. Visual aids simply are not on many people's radars or agency budgets, thus exploring the options and opportunities for the visual presentation of courtroom testimony is an oft-neglected tool in an attorney's or witness' toolbox. As a result, arguments and testimony are not always "sticking the landing" with some of those afore-mentioned tough crowds. Expert testimony may be diminished simply because a jury did not fully understand the case and its evidence when a few simple illustrations might have helped clarify key points.

Litigation graphics specialists leverage the principles of graphic design, com-munication, teaching, and even psychology to create visual aids that support a courtroom presentation or testimony, mindful of the fact that an effective visual aid can capture the jury's attention, invite their curiosity, and make complicated testimony clearer – all while simultaneously presenting an image of competence and authority. Simply put: a presentation with visual aids can make the presenter appear more concise, persuasive, and interesting than the same presenter giving the same presentation without visuals.

This chapter will emphasize the importance of visual aids during testimony, and demonstrate the utility of having a litigation graphics specialist on hand to help make courtroom presentations the most effective they can be. However, since not everyone has access to this type of support, this chapter also shares some basic principles that litigation graphics specialists use to polish presentations. The Forensic Anthropologist preparing for court can consider these principles and use them to make suggestions to the attorney regarding the best way to explain their findings to the jury. The conclusion of the chapter is a real world example where a litigation graphics specialist and Forensic Anthropologist worked together to create easy-to-understand supporting graphics for court testimony.

PowerPoint-style presentations are perhaps the most common types of visual aid used in court. The following elements should be considered when preparing or reviewing this type of aid.

## 10.1   Color

Color is one of the most basic elements of a presentation, and yet the one that can communicate the most. Color not only makes an image appealing or repellent, but can also give the viewer an impression about what they are seeing – not to mention an impression about the character of the person presenting.

The psychological and emotional effects of color (i.e. colors actually stirring or sedating various emotional states in people) is an interesting and controversial topic of study, but beyond the purview of this chapter. Being thoughtful about the use of color in its most basic ways, though, should be at the forefront of anyone's mind when making a visual presentation. One of these basic ways is simple legibility: color choices should make the visual aids easier, not harder, to view. Easy-to-see visuals have colors that are bold enough to stand out but not so vivid that they clash, make the image hard to see, or are difficult to look at for an extended period of time. The text should be in high contrast from the background. When unsure, it is always preferable to keep it simple and use black text on a white field or vice versa.

Another basic way to apply color is by considering traditional associations. If a color or colors are culturally or popularly linked to whatever is being depicted, that would be a traditional association. For example, with medical testimony exhibits with a "medical aesthetic" (mostly white with only soft, light blues, grays, or greens when color is needed) look more correct and appropriate to the average viewer, and thus more credible. Conversely, a slideshow of crime scene images might be more emotionally striking on a black background, but be cautious deviating much further: almost any solid color as a slide's background should generally be avoided unless very light.

This approach to color choices should be informed not only by the content of a presentation but the presenter themselves: a presentation from a law enforcement agency or university that wants to project an image of authority, experience, competence, and professionalism are not well represented by unconventional color choices. Traditional colors – as opposed to something a little too slick or trendy – will also hold up better should the case be re-evaluated during an appeals process years down the line. When in doubt, restraint and what seems "classic" is more likely to give an impression of confidence and seriousness.

## 10.2  Font

Consider the size of your display versus the distance the jury will sit from it, and choose a font size accordingly. If preparing for an unfamiliar courtroom, keep in mind the display could be 30–40 ft from the farthest juror. If a juror has to squint or strain to make out text, there is a very good chance it will not be read at all.

Avoid using unusual or novelty fonts – as with color, stick to the basics and use fonts that are clean, legible, and "standard." For most presentations, a font like Arial is a safe bet because it is easy to read and nearly universal (so there are no unexpected font substitutions when loading a presentation on a strange computer).

## 10.3  Layout

The concept of layout is fairly straightforward but worth explaining. Generally speaking, whatever is included on a slide (i.e. photos, video clips, or text) will look

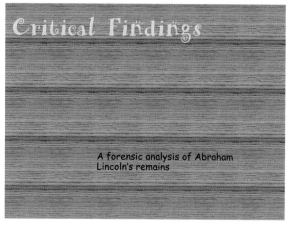

**Figure 10.1** An example of a trendy, cutesy, difficult-to-digest slide.

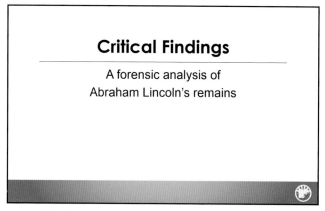

**Figure 10.2** An example of a clear, professional, easy-to-digest slide.

best centered both horizontally and vertically. This centering aids legibility and is one element that gives a presentation a professional and polished appearance (Figures 10.1 and 10.2).

A margin (1 in. is sufficient) should be present on all sides of a slide, so nothing is close to or extending past the slide's border. This margin also allows for situations where the display may not fully accommodate the image.

If using PowerPoint, there is a choice of slide formats. One format is 4:3 (closer to square), while the other is 16:9 ("widescreen"). Depending on the projection system or display device, one's slides could be "stretched" into the opposite ratio (e.g. a 4:3 slide could be stretched into a widescreen format by the courtroom's projector). Since one might be unfamiliar with the courtroom and its display equipment, creating slides in 4:3 is safer: square slides stretched wide are less distracting to look at than widescreen slides compressed into a square format, which can make text look extremely narrow and even illegible.

## 10.4   Clarity of purpose

The most common error in amateur presentations would be the lack of a clear purpose in a particular slide or even the presentation as a whole. Too often, presentations exist simply to give jurors something to look at other than the speaker. If there is no clear idea about what a visual aid is going to accomplish, it might not accomplish anything at all. Justify the existence of everything the jury will see, and be able to articulate the intent with each image. This exercise will actually help clarify and sharpen the argument or testimony.

Conversely, one should also be wary of overwhelming the viewer with information. Too much text is a frequent blunder. Slides with entire scanned documents or complete criminal statutes aren't appealing or inviting to look at (Figure 10.3).

How much text is acceptable for a single slide varies, but generally speaking one should err toward less, and the text should be emphasizing, summarizing, or highlighting what is being said – and not simply a transcription of every word being spoken. For example: on a presentation about the Pledge of Allegiance where it is recited out loud for the audience, it should not be written out word for word on a slide; a slide showing the title, "The Pledge of Allegiance," and perhaps significant words or phrases from the pledge appearing as they are spoken, would be more impactful.

## 10.5   The problem-solution approach to visual aids

Experts armed with these basic principles can now more effectively consider visual aids for their testimony. But how does one decide what to illustrate, and what to leave as unadorned testimony? One strategy is to approach the testimony using a "problem-solution" approach. Simply put, ask the following questions:
1. What are the most critical points or bits of information to convey to the jury?
2. What are the obstacles to the jury clearly understanding and retaining those critical points?
3. How could a visual aid minimize or negate those obstacles?
A few examples of this approach are given in the following.

A physician needs to testify about how the organs of the liver, stomach, pancreas, and spleen all fit together in the abdomen and where they are in relation to each another. The obstacle (or "problem") is that many of these organs are

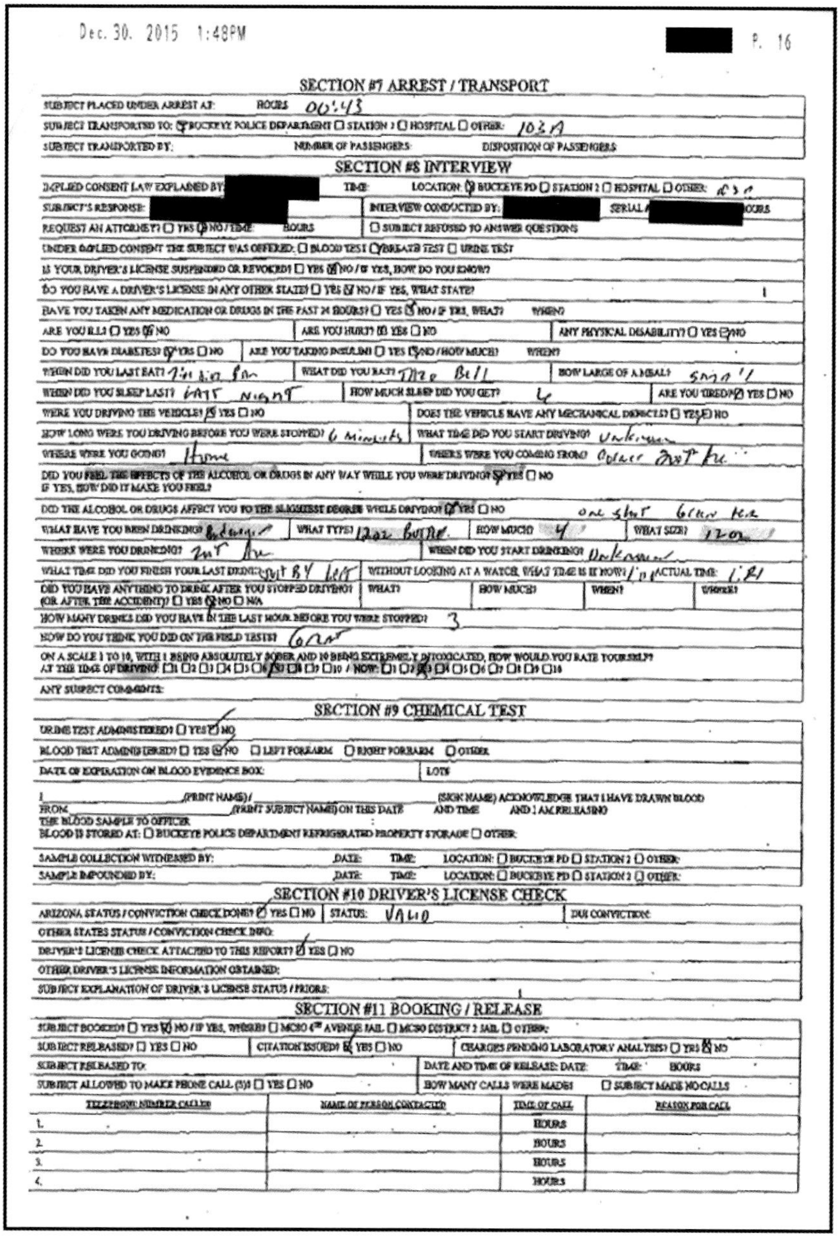

**Figure 10.3** An example of a scanned document that isn't legible or useful to viewers.

unfamiliar to the general public, they are unusual shapes, and they nest together rather than being simply side by side – thus challenging jurors to visualize their appearance and arrangement in their minds. The "solution" would be to create a simple illustration of the organs in question, semi-transparent so no organs are obscured and all clearly labeled, making the complexity of the testimony a non-issue. Another example would be having to explain to the jury how the defendant was the victim's half-cousin. Visualizing the closeness or distance of that relationship could be difficult for many (the problem). A family tree diagram removes that difficulty (solution). Another common problem that comes up in court is the description of a defendant's flight from officers. The verbal testimony about a pursuit of any length at all quickly devolves into a mind-numbing recitation of lefts, rights, and U-turns. A map of the overall area with a simple bright red arrow illustrating the route taken clarifies the sequence of events in the jurors' minds.

## 10.6 Case study

The best way to illustrate all of the concepts discussed and how they relate to forensic anthropological testimony is to share a real world example. What follows is a detailed description of a presentation created by the author in cooperation with a Forensic Anthropologist to aid her testimony in a criminal proceeding. By walking through the case's particulars, listing the issues to address with the presentation, and explaining the choices made in creating it, one will see more specifically how litigation graphics are created and used. The trial described below, *State of Arizona v. Avelino Tamala* (CR-2014005969), used visual aids to support the testimony of the Maricopa County Forensic Anthropologist, Dr. Laura Fulginiti.

On December 1, 1998, the partial skeletal remains of a child were found in the remote desert southwest of the Phoenix area. Sixteen years later, the remains were finally identified as "C.R.," age 3. Not long afterward, Avelino Guzman Tamala, a former boyfriend of the child's mother, was indicted.

Very little of C.R.'s skeleton was recovered: only a part of her skull (not quite two-thirds of her cranium), and even that little bit was shattered. Nevertheless, there was enough material present for Dr. Fulginiti to piece together the fragments and ultimately discern evidence of perimortem blunt force trauma – that is, fractures to the cranium around the time of death.

The first step is to consider all the obstacles inherent in presenting the critical facts to the jury. What does the jury need to know to understand the case and, of those things, which are potentially difficult to understand, follow, or retain? Viewing it from the problem-solution approach, the following obstacles would have to be overcome to make sure the jury was not only understanding the testimony Dr. Fulginiti would give, but would also find it persuasive:

1. *The average person's unfamiliarity with skeletal anatomy.* Most people know a skull when they see one – but when they are seeing one, it is most often a fake, complete, intact skull, viewed from certain angles, and in a movie. A real skull, a child's skull, and an incomplete one with none of the most recognizable landmarks (eye orbits, the nasal cavity, teeth, or a mandible) is far less recognizable. To complicate matters further, in this case the fragments had warped somewhat, introducing some asymmetry to what remained of the cranium. Even with a better-than-average knowledge of skulls and skeletal anatomy (with a degree in physical anthropology and being a former intern of Dr. Fulginiti), the author occasionally had to stop and reorient himself when handling C.R.'s remains to re-locate where her face would have been. As Dr. Fulginiti remarked throughout the process of photographing C.R.'s remains, "if *we* are having trouble orienting her cranium, then the jury is going to find it *especially* difficult."

2. *The visual and structural differences between fractures on "wet" (perimortem) versus "dry" (postmortem) bone.* Dr. Fulginiti was going to testify that specific fractures on a shattered partial cranium were characteristic of perimortem fractures. Like branches, bones break differently when they are wet/"green" versus dry. Those differences would have to be explained to a jury of laypeople who might not easily see the difference between one type of fracture versus another. If the distinction comes off as too subtle or perhaps only in the eye of the beholder a juror might find it difficult to appreciate – and therefore discount the testimony.

3. *Visualizing the fractures on multiple planes of the skull and visualizing the skull as a 3D shape.* Virtual 3D diagrams of crime scenes are often created so it is easier for jurors to visualize a space. Normal "2D" diagrams – the floorplans seen when looking at an apartment complex's brochure or a map of a zoo – are adequate for most viewers in most cases, but a significant portion of the population can find such diagrams very abstract. A floorplan has as much in common with a real space as the letter "A" has in common with the sound made when pronouncing it. A 2D diagram is not how the world is actually experienced, it is symbolic, and the symbol has to be "translated" in our minds into something meaningful. Some people are better at this than others. Complex anatomical shapes are no different: imagining how a skull would look from various angles would be challenging or impossible for some. If a juror cannot visualize a skull from a different perspective, he or she will certainly be incapable of imagining the directions from which someone was being struck.

4. *Viewing the remains not simply as fragments of bone but instead as C.R., a three-year-old child.* Also on the topic of abstraction is the concept that a scant

few fragments of bone that would barely fill a teacup are, in fact, the sole recovered remains of a child. What Dr. Fulginiti, the attorneys, the defendant and the jury will be looking at on the slides *is C.R.'s body*. In spending time talking about minute fractures and features on poker chip-sized pieces of bone, there is the risk of making the entire conversation academic and losing sight of that grim reality. How do we remind the jury, even subtly, that the case centers on a child victim?

Over the course of several weeks of office visits, Dr. Fulginiti and the author created and refined a PowerPoint presentation that would accompany her testimony. The process began with discussions about what her testimony would cover, what she felt the most important points were that she wanted to make, and what imagery would help her make those points. The cranial fragments were discussed, and photographed from many angles for use in the presentation. Dr. Fulginiti reviewed every major revision of the presentation and was able to suggest corrections, changes, or improvements. Once the presentation was nearly complete, it was "focus tested" with colleagues and the prosecuting attorneys. This testing garnered feedback that was used to further polish the presentation. By the time it was shown to the jury, it was as refined as possible and had everyone's confidence.

The final presentation began by showing the jury photographs of C.R.'s remains. To remind the jury that the bones were from a small child and not just miscellaneous specimens, almost every image of the fragments or reconstructed partial cranium was labeled with the child's name – not "fragments" or "bones" or even "remains."

Six views of the reconstructed cranium are shown on the second slide. As mentioned before, C.R.'s cranium was very incomplete and confusing to orient even for people with some knowledge of skeletal anatomy. To address this confusion, each view of the reconstructed fragments was superimposed over a line drawing of an intact, complete child's skull, to help viewers understand where the remains would be located in the head. Seeing all six views at once also suggests to the jury the notion of the skull as a 3D shape (Figure 10.4).

By the third slide, the presentation has begun to address three of the four major concerns identified before work began, just with two simple images and some carefully considered labeling.

The fourth slide addresses skull fractures. Before discussing the specifics of C.R.'s remains, an overview of the classic characteristics of skull fractures on "wet" bone was introduced to the jury. Titled "Characteristics of a Depressed Skull Fracture" (the type Dr. Fulginiti identified on this cranium), the slide shows the jury a simple line drawing of a child's skull. The image then animates how fractures develop and what they look like. While Dr. Fulginiti explained that linear fractures extend from the point of impact, the jury watched straight red

Recovered Fragments, Oriented

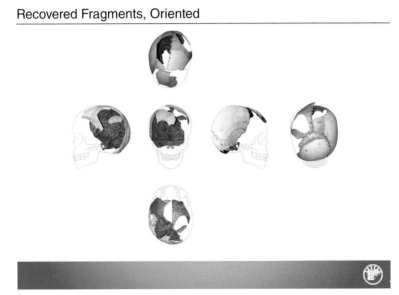

**Figure 10.4** Integration of the recovered fragments with a skull diagram.

lines growing outward from a point on the vault. When she explained that at some point the skull cannot flex inward any more before "failing" (fracturing), the jury watched sickle-shaped concentric fractures streak around the perimeter, drawing something like a bright red spider web on the side of the child's cranium (Figure 10.5).

The display is vivid, interesting to watch, and informative – and concludes in about eight seconds.

As said before, a jury is a "tough crowd." Experts have witnessed the rise of what author, professor, and social commentator Andrew Keen described as "the cult of the amateur" (Keen 2007). Experience, training, and credentials are not as powerfully persuasive as they once were. However distasteful we may find the notion, authority and expertise cannot be taken for granted as the beginning and end of persuasion. Dr. Fulginiti can describe her education and experience to a jury and then tell them "this is what I see in these remains" – but for some unknown percent of jurors, what might be even more effective is giving them the tools to be able to look at the evidence and decide they agree with her conclusion.

Now that the jury has walked through what a typical depressed skull fracture on wet bone looks like, the specifics of this case and this victim are brought back to the forefront, with the "classic" visual kept on screen as an exemplar to compare C.R.'s remains with. The next slide is a similar view of C.R.'s cranium (as with the second slide, superimposed over a line drawing of a complete skull so the jury can orient it), and via a series of highlights, labels, and simple

Characteristics of a Depressed Skull Fracture

Radial or concentric
fractures where bone
cracks inward

Linear fractures
extend from point
of impact

*Reference image: Berryman and Symes* 1998

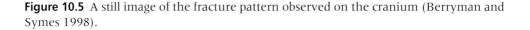

**Figure 10.5** A still image of the fracture pattern observed on the cranium (Berryman and Symes 1998).

animations, the presentation begins to call attention to the various features and damage visible on the bone as Dr. Fulginiti testifies to it. For example, a void removed for DNA analysis is shaded with a unique pattern. Different linear and concentric fractures are highlighted in vivid red lines, clearly drawing comparison with the identically rendered fractures on the exemplar beside it. This, explains Dr. Fulginiti, would be an impact. A second area is similarly highlighted and labeled as another impact, and the next slide moves to a different view of C.R.'s cranial vault to illustrate a third impact (Figure 10.6).

Every side of the victim's cranium is eventually reviewed, with impacts labeled in this manner (Figure 10.7).

Damage to her vault from rodent and carnivore activity is also pointed out and described, as well as damage from being exposed to the elements. The jury is walked through a methodical examination of the cranium, with clear photographs, diagrams, labels, and animations calling attention to whatever is being testified to in that particular moment. At one point, an unusual view of the cranium is shown, a three-quarter view from above, behind and to the left, to show stark discoloration between two adjacent, reassembled fragments. Dr. Fulginiti wanted to use the image to illustrate the difference between bones that were sun bleached for years versus buried – but the concern was whether the jury would understand what angle the cranium was being viewed from. To assist, a short animation of a virtual 3D skull viewed from the front (an orientation

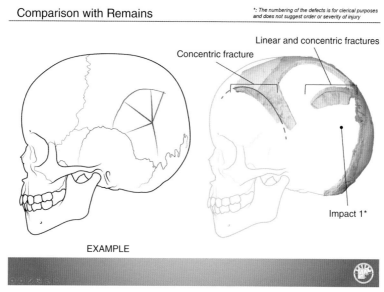

**Figure 10.6** Comparison of conceptual image with actual bone.

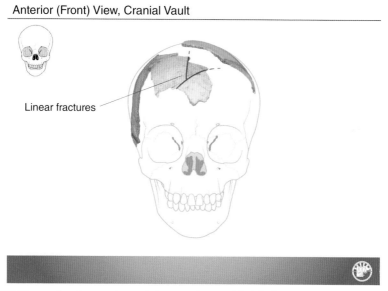

**Figure 10.7** Example of one view of the cranium with labeling.

most can immediately recognize) that then rotates into a position identical to the photograph is shown to help guide the viewer.

The final slide of the presentation set the images of the cranium aside entirely in favor of another 3D rendering, this time of a toddler. This aid was to serve three

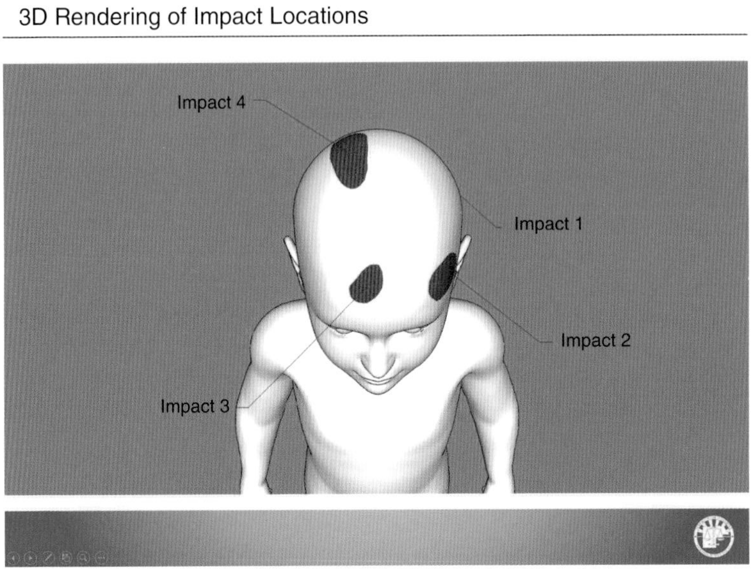

3D Rendering of Impact Locations

**Figure 10.8** Use of a 3D animated model to "humanize" the decedent for the jury.

purposes at once: first, to illustrate where exactly the impacts Dr. Fulginiti could identify were located on the victim's head. Secondly, to illustrate the improbability that the injuries could have been sustained shortly after death. (If the fractures occurred during burial, for example, when the grave was being tamped down, one would expect to see them all on one side of the head, not from virtually every angle.) And thirdly, to once again revisit the point that the fragments are not simply bits of bone, but were once living tissue in the head of a child (Figure 10.8).

According to Dr. Fulginiti and several other courtroom observers, the presentation was successful. Dr. Fulginiti – experienced with testifying in court, presenting, and teaching – noted jurors sat up, leaned forward and watched attentively when the slides were presented. They nodded when she would make rhetorical statements (e.g. "If you can see this right here … ") and took notes. Knowing one's testimony was effective is a win in and of itself, and often the only aspect a witness has any control over.

## 10.7  Conclusion

In a perfect world, jurors would be highly engaged in testimony, but there are a large number of other things potentially competing for their attention. To ensure that we are utilizing every option available to capture and hold that attention, communicating information effectively, and maximizing the odds they will retain it, visual aids that support arguments and testimony should be regarded as a normal part of any courtroom presentation or testimony. Thoughtfully prepared by an experienced litigation graphics specialist in cooperation with expert witnesses and attorneys, they can not only achieve those aims, but can increase the witness' own confidence and even understanding of the material about which they intend to testify. In the absence of a professional litigation graphic specialist, the expert can use the basic principles presented in this chapter to guide the graphics they will rely on during their testimony.

## References

Berryman, H.E. and Symes, S.A. (1998). Recognizing gunshot and blunt cranial trauma through fracture interpretation. In: *Forensic Osteology II: Advances in Identification of Human Remains* (ed. K. Reichs). Springfield, IL: C.C. Thomas.

Bigelow, J. and Poremba, A. (2014). Achilles' ear? Inferior human short-term and recognition memory in the auditory modality. *PLoS One* 9 (2): https://doi.org/10.1371/journal.pone.0089914.

Dscout. (2016). Mobile Touches: Dscout's Inaugural Study on Humans and Their Tech. Research report. https://blog.dscout.com/hubfs/downloads/dscout_mobile_touches_study_2016.pdf (accessed August 22, 2018).

Keen, A. (2007). *The Cult of the Amateur: How Today's Internet Is Killing our Culture*. New York, NY: Doubleday/Currency.

Schweitzer, N.J. and Saks, M.J. (2007). The CSI effect: popular fiction about forensic science affects public expectations about real forensic science. *Jurimetrics* 47: 357.

Shabiralyani, G., Hasan, K.S., Hamad, N., and Iqbal, N. (2015). Impact of visual aids in enhancing the learning process case research: district Dera Ghazi Khan. *Journal of Education and Practice* 6 (19): 226–233.

Vogel, D.R., Dickson, G.W., and Lehman, J.A. (1986). *Persuasion and the Role of Visual Presentation Support: The UM/3M Study*. Minneapolis, MN: Management Information Systems Research Center, School of Management, University of Minnesota.

## CHAPTER 11

# Maintaining independence in an adversarial system: expert witness testimony in forensic anthropology

Eric J. Bartelink[1], Laura C. Fulginiti[2], Alison Galloway[3], and Katherine M. Taylor[4]

[1] California State University, Chico, CA, USA
[2] Maricopa County, Office of the Medical Examiner, Phoenix, AZ, USA
[3] University of California, Santa Cruz, Santa Cruz, CA, USA
[4] King County Office of the Medical Examiner, Seattle, WA, USA

The adversarial nature of litigation makes it easy for experts to forget that they are not an advocate for one side or the other (Freckelton 2004; Hiss et al. 2007). Because anthropologists often receive substantial training in the study of the human condition, they may be inclined to show empathy and compassion for the decedents they study, which can sometimes interfere with objectivity. Scrutiny by a peer adds another layer of discomfiture to the process and if the peer is not someone known or implicitly trusted, those feelings can increase. Add to that the confounding variable of the manner in which attorneys discuss the opposing experts, particularly in informal contexts, and you have the setting for potentially awkward encounters. All of these factors can create hard feelings on one or both sides of any legal proceeding.

There are many important factors to consider when preparing for adversarial testimony. Most commonly, an opposing expert will be attached to the case with the hope that they will provide an alternative explanation for the findings. If there are no disagreements, the expert might look for flaws in the application of methodology or shortcomings in the handling of evidence. They might also comment on perceived over-interpretation, especially in trauma analysis. The expert performing the initial examination should prepare themselves for scrutiny and recognize that there will be limitations in any forensic analysis. Ego should be checked at the door, and instead the expert should try to learn from

*Forensic Anthropology and the United States Judicial System*, First Edition.
Edited by Laura C. Fulginiti, Kristen Hartnett-McCann, and Alison Galloway.
© 2019 John Wiley & Sons Ltd. Published 2019 by John Wiley & Sons Ltd.

criticisms, especially if they result in improvements to their future casework. First and foremost, the experts on both sides should try to remember that they are not responsible for any categorizations made by the attorneys. The attorneys may not fully comprehend the findings and thus misstate or misrepresent an expert's opinion. The attorneys, contrary to the experts, are advocates and will interpret the findings in a way that more advantageously supports their theory of the case (Weinstock et al. 2003).

Another important consideration for the expert brought in to review someone else's work is context. Often a significant amount of time has passed since the original examination and methods or interpretations may have evolved. Similarly, the examining expert may have been compromised by procedures applied to their examination from the agency who requested it. There may have been other intangible factors at play that do not come out in the crossfire between the two sides. The second expert should caveat their report with recognition of these potential influencing factors.

One of the authors has now had interactions with seven of her peers, two of them on multiple occasions. Each of these interactions carried "lessons learned" moments. She and her mentor Dr. Walter Birkby were on opposite sides twice, both at times when his health prevented him from being able to defend himself or his work. She has been on the opposite side of five individuals she considers to be friends. Each of these encounters provoked different feelings among the experts. For two of them there was rancor and discord and for three of them there were no repercussions and life went on as before the process. In those latter instances, all of the experts seemed to recognize that the process is adversarial but that the experts do not have to be (Weinstock et al. 2003). The lessons learned include: that the Forensic Anthropologist cannot control what the "opposing" expert thinks or says about them outside of the courtroom; that an expert cannot control how the work is characterized by the opposing attorney; that an expert only controls their own demeanor in the face of these experiences; and objectivity is the rule of the day. The Forensic Anthropologist is not an advocate for one side or the other; nor are they an advocate for the victim. Forensic Anthropologists are responsible for providing reliable, science-based observations as they apply to the cause and manner being determined by the medical examiner, to the scientific identification of the decedent, or to matters of time since death and the scene of recovery (Galloway et al. 1990).

When a Forensic Anthropologist is the reviewing expert they are responsible for examining the methodology behind the findings, commenting on the reliability or scientific underpinnings of any interpretations of the findings, and dissecting out where there might be shortcomings in how the findings were achieved. The review is not a personal attack. The expert on the opposing side should not be seen as the enemy, or incompetent, or lazy. They are human beings, capable of making mistakes but also capable of learning from them and adjusting as necessary. One may have more pertinent experience than the other or one may have more research background in a subject than the other. Who to believe is up to the jury or the judge and it should not reflect back on the two experts or their ongoing relationship.

In many jurisdictions, opposing experts typically do not communicate with one another during their evaluation of the evidence. This communication can vary but many attorneys prefer independent examinations, and in fact, the legal system has processes in place to preclude communication (Federal Rules of Evidence, Rule 615). In some cases, the opposition's expert might be present during the examination as an observer only. During these actions both experts should be aware that any comments made, or opinions shared, are subject to discovery by the other side. The interaction should be kept professional, without personal kibitzing or trivial conversation. That does not mean the experts have to be stoic or unfriendly toward one another. Once the examination is complete the experts do not have the luxury of comparing notes or discussing the findings until the trial is concluded. In some instances, the Judge may not lift "the rule" until the appeals process is complete, although this is rare.

Often, the only "communication" between two experts is by affidavit or through the deposition process. A deposition is a formal type of interview garnering sworn testimony that is typically audio and/or video recorded (see Chapter 9). Once the deposition is concluded, the expert will be given an opportunity to review the transcript and make any corrections or clarifications. These can be as minor as typos or misspellings, or as major as not being allowed to adequately explain an important concept. The expert should always take the time to request and review the deposition transcript and submit any changes promptly. Usually there is a deadline associated with the return of the comments and it must be met. For some expert interactions, a candid discussion at the conclusion of the legal process is enlightening and helpful. Mischaracterizations by the attorneys can be discussed and usually any residual resentment can be hammered out. All scientists should be able to confer and improve their skill set by comparison with others. These conversations provide the means to move the discipline forward and to raise one another up instead of putting each other down.

## 11.1 Criminal vs. civil cases

Although Forensic Anthropologists are more likely to testify in criminal cases than civil cases, their expertise plays a similar role regardless. Criminal cases almost always involve homicide, and the Forensic Anthropologist may be called in to testify about scene recovery, biological profile, personal identification, and most commonly, perimortem skeletal trauma (Lesciotto 2015). In both criminal and civil cases, the opposing counsel may request the services of another Forensic Anthropologist, who may conduct a case review of records and sometimes an independent skeletal analysis (Galloway et al. 1990). While this may appear to place the opposing experts in an adversarial position, the experts should view this as a series of checks and balances. If both experts are committed to scientific integrity and ethical practice, the testimony may provide a more nuanced understanding of the strengths and limitations of the science to the jury.

While Forensic Anthropology testimony may include discussion of the biological profile and antemortem conditions, the decedent will almost always have been positively identified prior to the trial. Thus, for criminal cases the Forensic Anthropologist's testimony most often focuses on skeletal findings to support the cause and manner of death, such as evidence of perimortem trauma (Lesciotto 2015).

The report must provide extensive documentation of skeletal trauma, including descriptions, photographs, diagrams, measurements, and bench notes (see Chapters 6 and 7). Because these data are discoverable by the other side, experts are expected to share their documentation with the opposing counsel. Forensic Anthropologists should be prepared to defend their conclusions and should anticipate limitations and areas of weakness in the analysis, whether dictated by the science, availability of scientific equipment, limitations based on the specific nature of case (e.g. skeletal preservation and completeness), or other factors. Given the high stakes in a criminal homicide trial, Forensic Anthropologists should stay within their scope of expertise, be careful not to over-interpret skeletal findings, and avoid potentially inflammatory language.

Civil cases often involve litigation regarding the identity or condition of human remains, and unlike criminal cases, almost always involve a request for some form of financial compensation by the plaintiff. Common disputes include misplaced, switched, or contaminated cremains, the loss of skeletal elements during transfers of remains between cemeteries, illegal disposal of remains by cemeteries or tissue banks, and the state of preservation of a body at the time of funeral. These cases often involve large lawsuits for damages, ranging from thousands of dollars to even millions of dollars. More rarely, wrongful death suits can be brought in cases where the criminal trial either yields a not guilty verdict, or the plaintiff seeks monetary compensation for the loss independent of the criminal proceedings. Forensic Anthropologists should be aware of the dynamics of a civil trial, especially given that the plaintiff's attorneys will be seeking maximum damages. Further, they should not be surprised by the intensity of the adversarial process, which often exceeds that of criminal cases. The expert should also make it clear to attorneys from the start of their involvement that they will only report on findings that can be scientifically demonstrated, regardless of whether or not it supports their case.

## 11.2   Courtroom roles and rules

The prosecution's role in a criminal case is to present evidence of a crime as it pertains to the individual on trial. They serve as a voice for the community and as an advocate of the victim, acting as both a government attorney and a government representative (e.g. district attorney's officer). They are expected to coordinate with law enforcement in the investigation of crimes, to determine whether there is sufficient evidence to go to trial, and to serve as an attorney during legal proceedings. In contrast, the defense's role is to serve as an advocate to the defendant, protecting their interests by ensuring that any evidence is supported by fact and by rigorous investigation of any claims or findings presented by the prosecution. The unbalanced nature of the US legal system often puts the defense at a disadvantage, especially in cases where the defendant is represented by a public defender. The public defender is appointed by the court to represent a defendant and often lacks the same level of financial resources granted to prosecutors. This disadvantage may hinder the defense's ability to obtain forensic experts to oppose the prosecution's experts. Typically, the public defender must take the matter to the court to obtain permission to retain and fund the services of an expert witness prior to any work being conducted. However, if a defendant is able to afford their own legal counsel, they are at less of a disadvantage than if they use a public defender.

Judges play a central role in both criminal and civil trials. They are tasked with the role of interpreting the law. They manage the trial, maintain order in the courtroom, act as a referee between opposing counsel, rule on motions, weigh the facts of a case (for non-jury trials), protect the trial against biasing or inadmissible information, and often dictate the sentence for the convicted defendant. The judge also determines whether an individual has the appropriate credentials to offer an expert opinion in the case and then ensures that expert witnesses are properly sworn in and dismissed from the stand. If an expert witness' statements are challenged by the opposing counsel, the judge may rule whether or not statements can be admitted, or struck from the record.

In both criminal and civil trials, legal and medico-legal experts each have their role to play in the trial or legal deposition. While not expected to have a deep understanding of law, Forensic Anthropologists should be cognizant of their role in a case, as well as the role of other experts, the attorneys for the prosecution and the defense, and the judge and jury. The adversarial nature of court trials can be a shock to experts who may be used to more cordial environments, such as academia, where direct confrontation is often avoided in favor of more circumspect methods. Attorneys on both sides may leave little room for nuance and uncertainty, and expect expert witnesses to provide cut and dried responses. For experts who rarely testify, the process can be disconcerting, especially if they need to qualify certain findings (e.g. uncertainty in determination of perimortem trauma vs. postmortem damage).

The expert must re-familiarize themselves with the case prior to trial, including a comprehensive review of the report, bench notes, photographs, and deposition statements (see Chapter 9). Often the attorneys who requested the expert's services will conduct a pretrial review of the case to make sure there is common understanding of the pertinent findings and also to aid with preparing the case for trial. The expert should present non-technical explanations of key findings in a language that can be understood by a jury. Analogies can be helpful to facilitate understanding of concepts, as well as using more general terminology than that provided in the case report. Juries often comprise a range of backgrounds and education, so there should be no assumption of a certain level of technical understanding of scientific methods. The expert may be asked to use a pointer or "draw" on a computer screen to identify skeletal features or trauma in photographs or diagrams for the jury, which is an effective method for describing skeletal findings.

During direct and cross examination, attorneys may ask open-ended, multi-part or complex, and/or convoluted questions that are difficult to follow or answer. The expert should be prepared to ask them to reduce a multi-part question into single questions, or to restate a question in a less tortuous manner (see Chapter 9). Similarly, attorneys will ask the same question in a variety of ways hoping to elicit a different response or to push an expert into contradicting themselves. Careful listening and maintaining patience while explaining again to the jury is critical in these situations.

Finally, Forensic Anthropologists should anticipate being asked questions outside their scope of expertise. The opposing counsel may ask questions pertaining to other aspects of the case, either due to their lack of understanding of different forensic specialties or as an attempt to discredit an expert who takes the bait. Often these questions pertain to interpretation of soft tissue injuries or cause and manner of death, which are all within the scope of the forensic pathologist or medical examiner. By anticipating all these types of questions, Forensic Anthropologists should feel comfortable answering "that question is outside the scope of my expertise" or asking for a restatement of the question(s).

## 11.3   Case studies

Forensic Anthropologists work in a wide variety of settings and not all will testify during their careers. Given that little published literature is available on expert witness confrontation, each co-author contributed a case study outlining unanticipated issues between experts and how they were handled. These case studies also highlight the importance of maintaining professionalism when defending your work, addressing criticism from opposing counsel, or when reviewing the work of other experts.

### 11.3.1   Case study 1

The skeletal remains of three teenage females and a fetus were recovered from a 50 ft deep, earthen well. The decedents were deposited in the well in the mid-1980s by a serial killer duo responsible for multiple homicides. Despite being convicted of several of these homicides, one of the co-defendants had his life sentence reduced to 14 years due to a technicality. His early parole caused the other co-defendant much angst, given that he received a death sentence. A bounty hunter advocating for victims' families offered a large sum of money to the death row inmate in return for hand drawn maps identifying the burial site locations of several homicide victims that were never recovered. After being notified of these maps, the parolee committed suicide fearing incarceration for his role in additional homicides. The maps were released to the press and to the sheriff-coroner, unleashing a media frenzy. Despite the sensationalized media coverage, these developments provided hope to families waiting for answers.

The sheriff's office proceeded hastily on the recovery efforts, and did not request the services of either a Forensic Anthropologist or archeologist. The remains of two human skeletons were recovered from a property owned by one of the convicted men's family; however, the defendants had previously been tried and convicted of these "no body" homicides. The sheriff's office next turned their attention to the map identifying the location of the earthen well provided by the death row inmate. The well was located along a rural road and had been filled in with soil and debris by the landowner long after the homicides took place. No Forensic Anthropologist or archeologist had been requested for the scene. The sheriff's office opted to excavate the well using large earth moving equipment, including a bulldozer and a long-armed backhoe with a toothed-bucket. The backhoe was used to create several piles of soil and debris, which were sifted by crime scene personnel over the course of a week. The sheriff's office quantified the success of the excavation to the media based on the number of bone fragments recovered, which eventually exceeded 1700 pieces. In a moment of irony, a sheriff's office spokesperson stated that they planned to bring in an archeologist to assist *after* they had recovered all human remains from the well. Local media obtained and broadcasted close-up photographs of the soil piles, human remains, personal effects, and forensic evidence, as well as aerial photographs of the remains and evidence laid out on the sorting tables.

Once remains and evidence were sorted, the sheriff's office reached out to an anthropologist from a local university to assist with the analysis of the remains. The destructive nature of the excavation presented challenges for skeletal analysis, including a high level of fragmentation, extensive commingling, and an unknown number of victims. The anthropologist was tasked with sorting the commingled remains, generating biological profiles, and documenting other identifying characteristics. Within a short period of time, two of the three teenage decedents were identified through dental records and DNA testing. However, the third victim, a pregnant female, has yet to be identified. In the weeks following the analysis, the remains of the two identified females were returned to next of kin.

The family of one of the identified victims expressed concerns regarding the completeness and integrity of the remains they received, given the use of earth moving equipment in the recovery effort. With the help of the family's attorney and a retired law enforcement officer, the remains were released to one of the authors for analysis and to evaluate for possible commingling. The remains were jumbled within a child-sized body bag, and thus were not sorted or bagged by element. Early in the analysis, it was clear that there was duplication of numerous elements indicating commingling. In addition, a fetal innominate was also located with the remains, presumably belonging to the unidentified female's fetus. The skeletal elements were identified and sorted to conduct a comprehensive inventory and analysis. Commingling was determined based on anatomical duplication, size discrepancies between bilateral elements, and inconsistency in overall size with the decedent's known remains. The majority of the remains were consistent with the identified decedent; however, the analysis revealed a minimum of 28 commingled elements from at least three different individuals as well as the additional fetal bone. The victim's diminutive body size in comparison with the other two victims aided significantly in sorting the remains, especially for determining which commingled elements were most likely from one of the other two victims.

Commingled remains included fragments of cranial vault, facial bones, a first cervical vertebra, a radius, a humerus, several metacarpals and hand phalanges, several metatarsals, two ilium fragments, and several ribs. DNA testing further established that one of the commingled skeletal elements belonged to the other identified female. Because the opposing anthropologist's report was initially unavailable, it was difficult to determine whether commingling resulted from the recovery efforts, the anthropological analysis, or both.

Based on the author's findings, the family's attorney filed a civil lawsuit against the sheriff's office and the county for negligence in the recovery efforts and subsequent handling of the decedent's remains. Attorneys representing both the county and victim's family deposed several experts, including the author and the original anthropologist. The opposing attorney was required to provide the original Forensic Anthropology report to the author just prior to the deposition. Although the opposing anthropologist and author had no prior interactions, the deposition was clearly designed for confrontation between the experts. During the nearly two-hour deposition, the opposing attorney questioned the author on bone identifications and how commingling was established in an attempt to discredit the report.

Although the opposing attorney was very aggressive during the deposition, the author focused on what could be scientifically demonstrated from the skeletal analysis and report. Several attempts were made to discredit the findings, however the analysis was extensively documented through numerous labeled photographs and descriptions embedded in the report. Navigating this complex case was a challenge not for only the author, but for all involved experts and attorneys. In both criminal and civil cases, Forensic Anthropologists should be prepared for aggressive questioning and ad hominem (directed at the person rather than at the position they are taking) attacks by opposing attorneys. When asked to evaluate the work of other anthropologists, the expert should focus on the scientific content of the report, and not launch into criticism of the expert.

Lessons learned: There were several lessons learned during the analysis and subsequent deposition of this case. The author's involvement in these legal proceedings was instructive as it provided a more in-depth perspective of the dynamics of civil cases and how attorneys may attempt to distort information provided in expert witness reports. The ability to maintain composure during an intense two-hour deposition was crucial, and ultimately led to a more cordial interaction with the opposing attorney. Repetition is helpful as well as providing explanations of the same thing in multiple ways to clarify points, especially to attorneys that may have limited knowledge of Forensic Anthropology.

### 11.3.2   Case study 2

Approaching a case from the perspective of the expert retained by the defense can be challenging. We are immediately embedded in an attack strategy and the emotions that are produced can quickly engulf both sides. In a case involving the death of a woman whose skeletonized remains were recovered a considerable period of time after her death, one author was retained by the defense to assess the report of the Forensic Anthropologist who conducted the initial findings. The initial request was to assess the report and any weaknesses that should be questioned.

In the course of examination of the available material, a sharp division of interpretation became clear. One expert ascribed injuries to the anterior ribs as perimortem fracturing due to homicidal actions – either stomping or crushing actions to the chest. The expert retained by the defense attributed these same defects as a combination of sharp force trauma along with fracturing and occurring during the postmortem period. This damage was deemed consistent with the actions of the pathologist, as reported in the autopsy report, of opening the rib cage during the postmortem examination. What had started as a basic review quickly necessitated a re-examination of the bones at the home base of the expert retained by the prosecution. Arrangements were made for the anthropologist and the pathologist, both retained by the defense, to examine the skeletal material that was still housed at the original anthropologist's facilities.

When another anthropologist is examining bones in the course of preparation of a case for the defense, the prosecution usually insists on being present to prevent any alteration or loss of the material. Typically, one to two people will be present and watching throughout the re-examination period. In this particular case, a lesson in etiquette in such situations quickly developed. The prosecution team was relatively large, milled around the examination area and chatted loudly making the work by the two defense experts difficult. Some basic lessons from this experience are (i) that the examining expert(s) should request ahead of time that the prosecution team and their expert are permitted only to observe from a distance and may not approach or try to intimidate or use this time as a second chance to review the case, (ii) that the examining team should be allowed to converse in low tones without being overheard, and (iii) the attending parties should not create conditions where the visiting experts cannot focus on their work. All parties have the right to expert opinions, whether or not those opinions help in the case. The decision to include that information lies with the defendant and their attorneys. The examining expert should take the time to lay out the conditions under which they wish to conduct their examination prior to agreeing to review the case.

After other convolutions, this case did proceed to trial and resulted in the conviction of the defendant. As often happens with cases in which there are sharply divergent opinions, both experts were asked to come to court at the same time so that any rebuttal could be handled in one period of time. Whatever the previous negative interactions between experts, these should not be brought forward during the testimony nor in discussions in the courtroom. There is an exception to "the rule" that allows expert witnesses to be present in the courtroom while the other expert is testifying. While this can be uncomfortable, the opportunity to hear directly from the other Forensic Anthropologist can be very helpful when trying to assess their opinion.

The trial also brought with it another tactic that may be encountered by those going to court – the "on-the-spot" challenge. In this case, a set of pig rib bones had been prepared by the expert retained by the prosecution, some that were fractured and others partially cut and then snapped. These bones were handed to the defense expert on the witness stand to assess how many of each were in the set. With limited time on the stand in which to do this, a quick assessment was made, an answer provided, and the prosecuting attorney very quickly moved on to another topic. The defense expert assumed that the answer must have been correct.

Lessons learned: Often a medical examiner, coroner or district attorney's office will enforce policies limiting the examination by forensic scientists hired by opposing counsel. This limitation may affect the duration of observation, the number of times material can be viewed and who is present during the observation. Before progressing to an examination, these ground rules should be clear. Ideally, the specimens are monitored by a morgue staff person without knowledge of the case to avoid any contamination. Other members of the team, such as the pathologist, should document important features during the examination time but conversations about the findings are best left for a time when there is no outside person to overhear.

### 11.3.3   Case study 3

Two cases are compared here with regard to expert witness interactions: one positive, and one negative. In the first, a young woman was discovered in the den of her home amidst evidence of a struggle. Blood pools and spatter were numerous and furniture was displaced. At the autopsy the pathologist discovered that the cranial vault had sustained major damage and was fragmented into several pieces. The Forensic Anthropologist was asked to perform a reconstruction of the skull and interpret the defects. During the course of the investigation a particular implement was alleged to have produced the damage to the vault. The Forensic Anthropologist included a comment regarding that implement in the report after assessing it in the context of the injuries.

As the case wended its way to trial there were numerous pretrial meetings and interviews. During the first pretrial interview, the first question asked of the Forensic Anthropologist was whether they were going to opine that the implement caused the injuries. The attorney made it clear that his expert had told him that the injuries could not be narrowed down to a single implement. The Forensic Anthropologist indicated that the proffered opinion would be that the implement could not be ruled out but that it was not the only possible cause of the observed injuries. As the interview proceeded more questions that clearly came from the defense expert were asked. The answers appeared to stymie the attorney but much of his bluster faded as he realized that the Forensic Anthropologist for the State was far more objective than he had been led to believe.

The prosecuting attorney later advised the Forensic Anthropologist that an expert had been retained by the defense which dovetailed with the impression at the interview. This defense expert was very familiar to the author and was some-one both respected and admired. The defense expert had in fact been a large part of the author's formative training. The defense attorney used that information to attempt to undermine the author's confidence and to impugn the methods used by the author. For example, the defense expert told the defense attorney that the report should include the traditional six view drawings of the trauma. As a result, the attorney made a request to the author to produce these drawings. He seemed convinced that it could not be done. The author explained that those diagrams had not been created because there were so many fractures and the photographs of the skull captured them in a much more manageable manner. However, after the request, the diagrams were produced. (The defense expert later confided that all of the photographs obtained by the original Forensic Anthropologist were not provided to them for review).

The intimidation continued at trial as the defense attorney had a series of questions that were clearly the results of his conversations with the retained expert. They were detailed and focused in a way that most cross-examinations are not. This allowed the author to clearly and definitively describe the scientific findings to the jury. By providing instruction to the attorney, the retained expert had actually made the job of the original Forensic Anthropologist much easier. In the end, they did not disagree about the cause of the injuries or the mechanism.

During the build-up to the trial, the American Academy of Forensic Sciences meeting took place. The two experts were at dinner together and the case came up in conversation. The retained expert simply said "well, we are not going to discuss that right now" and that was the end of it. The relationship is intact; the respect is still fully evident and the science was allowed to speak for itself.

Contrast this example with another case involving a young woman who was found deceased in similar circumstances. In this particular case the retained expert was fed false and misleading information regarding the science and became quite hostile to the original Forensic Anthropologist. These two experts had also known each other for many years and had tremendous respect for one another. The defense attorney engaged in ad hominem attacks and he embroiled the retained expert in them rather than concentrating on the findings. By the time the trial was concluded the two experts were not on speaking terms. This was not the fault of the experts, but rather the result of an attorney who was willing to distort the science and the facts of the case in order to solicit a favorable verdict. In these instances, the experts must be able to focus on the evidence and avoid becoming embroiled in the "winning" or "losing" contest.

Our job as experts is to provide reliable interpretation of bony injuries based on strong underlying science. We are not advocates. And, more importantly, we work in a very small discipline where our paths are going to continue to cross. Professionalism, collegiality, and respect must dictate our actions.

Lessons learned: The discipline of Forensic Anthropology is small and most practitioners either know one another very well or have name recognition. Rather than being intimidated, or anxious, or rancorous and disrespectful the practitioner should use these situations to improve their techniques and methods, to put science to the test and to allow the court to hear unbiased, unemotional facts regarding sometimes complicated, technical information. The experts who oppose one another should remain cordial rather than buying into the idea that they are advocating for one side or the other and behaving accordingly.

### 11.3.4   Case study 4

A young female was found dead at her residence and her caregivers charged with homicide by neglect. As the case approached trial, the documented age of the decedent became a focal issue for the case. Under state law, homicide by neglect was only applicable if the decedent was 16 or younger. If she was over 16 years of age, the charge was manslaughter by neglect. Because the decedent was born in a foreign country that did not generate birth certificates, there was no official documentation of her year of birth. In an effort to resolve the issue, the decedent was exhumed and radiographs were obtained to facilitate an age estimation based on skeletal and dental maturation. The state's Forensic Anthropologist informed the prosecutor from the onset that given the reported age of the decedent, the age range resulting from radiographic analysis was likely to include the age of 16, and in fact it did.

The defense hired a radiologist to perform an independent assessment of the images. The radiologist examined the radiographs taken by the author and reviewed their Forensic Anthropology report. The radiologist was not familiar to the author and there was no interaction between the two experts beyond each reading the other's reports. The radiologist provided his own age-at-death based on the radiographs.

Testimony during the trial was complicated by the physical configuration of the courtroom. The courtroom had two rows of large windows, and blinds for the lower row only. The upper, unreachable row could not be covered. On the day the author testified there was bright sunshine and the courtroom was very bright. The jury understandably had difficulty seeing fine detail in the projected radiographs. Under questioning by the State, the author was able to provide detailed information regarding juvenile bone growth and how to differentiate between the different phases of growth on a radiograph.

Contrariwise, on the day the defense expert testified, the weather was overcast and conditions were far more preferable for viewing a projected radiograph. The prosecutor related to the author that he challenged the defense expert on his interpretation of skeletal maturity by projecting a magnified radiograph that was easily visible given the improved lighting conditions. When challenged, the defense expert reportedly attacked the credibility of the author rather than concede that the radiograph did not support his opinion. When the author was called again as a rebuttal witness, the defense tried to discredit them by pointing out that their degree is "in philosophy." While a common distractor for testimony is to discredit by claiming Forensic Anthropologists are not medical or "real" doctors, claiming the degree was in philosophy demonstrated either gross ignorance of the degree process, or a deliberate attempt to obfuscate. In either case, the Forensic Anthropologist was able to refute the statement easily by stating "yes, that is what a PhD is, regardless of the discipline."

Although the prosecutor expressed dismay at the portrayal of the Forensic Anthropologist by the defense expert, the author was able to take it in their stride understanding that ad hominem attacks generally mean the science does not support the theory of the case they are presenting. The author also knows that the role of the Forensic Anthropologist is not to convince the jury that one viewpoint is correct, but rather to give them the tools to understand how they reached his or her conclusion so that they can decide on the validity of the evidence. The underlying irony throughout the testimony was that the Forensic Anthropologist's age range did not exclusively support the assertions of either side because the age range spanned the crucial age of 16.

Lessons learned: A Forensic Anthropologist called by the prosecution can be called back as a rebuttal witness when the defense hires their own expert. That expert does not have to be another Forensic Anthropologist, but may instead be a medical doctor. Attacks on the credibility and qualifications of the Forensic Anthropologist can be part of the defense strategy and should not rattle the anthropologist. The job of the anthropologist is to testify to his or her findings, independent of what another expert proposes and regardless of any personal attacks by opposing council.

## 11.4   Conclusion

Forensic Anthropologists should be prepared for the adversarial nature of court trials and other legal proceedings, regardless of whether it is a criminal or civil trial or by which side they have been retained. They should never advocate for one side or the other, or for the victim, and instead should focus on their role as an expert who provides reliable and science-based observations. Further, when reviewing the work of other forensic experts, keeping the focus on the analysis and the methods rather than ad hominem attacks is critical. Maintaining professionalism in these circumstances can be difficult, especially when the quality of the work is being challenged, or when the emotions of the interested parties run high. Nevertheless, all experts should strive for objectivity even under such demanding circumstances.

## References

Freckelton, I. (2004). Regulating forensic deviance: the ethical responsibilities of expert report writers and witnesses. *Journal of Law and Medicine* 12 (2): 141–149.

Galloway, A., Birkby, W.H., Kahana, T., and Fulginiti, L. (1990). Physical anthropology and the law: legal responsibilities of Forensic Anthropologists. *American Journal of Physical Anthropology* 33 (S11): 39–57.

Hiss, J., Freund, M., and Kahana, T. (2007). The forensic expert witness – an issue of competency. *Forensic Science International* 168 (2–3): 89–94.

Lesciotto, K.M. (2015). The impact of Daubert on the admissibility of Forensic Anthropology expert testimony. *Journal of Forensic Sciences* 60 (3): 549–555.

Weinstock, R., Leong, G.B., and Silva, J.A. (2003). Ethical guidelines. In: *Principles and Practice of Forensic Psychiatry*, 2e (ed. R. Rosner), 56–72. London: Arnold.

## CHAPTER 12

# Valuing your time: appropriate calculation of fees and expenses as an expert witness

Alison Galloway[1], Eric J. Bartelink[2], and Kristen Hartnett-McCann[3]

[1] *University of California, Santa Cruz, Santa Cruz, CA, USA*
[2] *California State University, Chico, CA, USA*
[3] *State of Connecticut, Office of the Chief Medical Examiner, Farmington, CT, USA*

One area in Forensic Anthropology with little guidance is the compensation that the expert witness/Forensic Anthropologist should receive for the time devoted to a case. Serving as an expert witness and testifying in court are not typically part of formal training, even in graduate programs in Forensic Anthropology. The complexities of this topic come not from the concept of charging for the time but the competing contexts of the legal realm and responsibilities that many anthropologists hold to their regular employer. Beyond discussion of some obvious errors in charging, few guides for expert witnesses provide information on how to structure fees, what can and cannot be charged, and when payment is due. How to separate a business entity from an institutional identity is also an issue for many anthropologists who work in an educational institution or a government forensic sciences laboratory.

In the following sections, this chapter addresses the historic foundations of expert witness compensation, fees for services rendered, and the situations in which an expert may choose not to charge for work. Recommendations and guidance are provided for reasonable expenses, invoicing, and establishing agreements for fee-based services. This chapter does not discuss salary amounts for full or part time employment.

*Forensic Anthropology and the United States Judicial System*, First Edition.
Edited by Laura C. Fulginiti, Kristen Hartnett-McCann, and Alison Galloway.
© 2019 John Wiley & Sons Ltd. Published 2019 by John Wiley & Sons Ltd.

## 12.1   History of expert witnesses and compensation

The history of fees charged by witnesses begins with the development of the expert witness as distinct from the role of the lay witness, the evolution of both the prosecution and defense developing a "case" for presentation to the jury and for attorneys taking over the questioning of witnesses. These transitions occurred around the mid-1700s in the United States and Great Britain (Golan 1999, 2008) and set the expert witness apart as a separate and distinct entity in the courtroom.

One of the early instances of expert witnesses appearing in court was the Wells Harbor case (*Folkes v. Chadd*) in England in 1782 (Golan 1999, 2008). This civil trial presented paid expert witnesses on the topic of tidal flow and sediment accumulation in a harbor against claims that a specific embankment was to blame. Experts had previously appeared in court prior to that case but were largely court-nominated rather than being retained by one side of the argument.

By the middle of the 1800s, serving as a scientist in court had become a lucrative means of supplementing income (Golan 1999, 2008). In Great Britain, the friction this produced was exacerbated by the class structure as science shifted from a "gentleman's" hobby to a career achievable to men who could obtain sufficient education. By the end of the century, the battles between competing experts caused great confusion among judges and juries and the conclusion was often that all such testimony was highly suspect (Graham 1977).

In the early 1900s, the friction over expert witness payments resulted in some jurisdictions being willing to compel testimony from experts without the right for compensation beyond normal witness fees (Morgan 1953). This approach seriously disadvantaged the indigent party, making it difficult to retain any expert willing to provide insight on their case.

## 12.2   Models of compensation

In modern courts, expert witnesses are required to appear in person to support the scientific arguments provided. As a consequence, the acceptance of fees as compensation for the time required to develop an opinion and to testify to that opinion in court is now widely accepted as standard practice. The relevant services covered would include the time acquiring the case and documentation, completing the chain of custody, producing the intake documentation, cleaning and securely storing the material, conducting the analysis and imaging of the remains, calculation of any metric and morphoscopic analyses, and production of the final report. Additional costs will be incurred if and when the case goes to trial and are usually considered as a separate suite of expenses from the case itself. There may be pretrial interviews, depositions, informal conversations or meetings and all time, including preparation for these, must be documented for financial recompense. In large part, this is due to both the infrequent nature of cases proceeding to trial and the length of time between the examination and the testimony.

### 12.2.1   Retainers

A retainer is the fee paid to an expert to secure their services. A retainer mitigates the risk to the expert and can be a significant amount, often a large portion of the potential earnings from a case. The fees accrued during the course of the analysis, pretrial processes, and testimony in court are charged against the retainer as the case progresses. The client may be (and often is) required to replenish the retainer from time to time. A portion of the retainer may be deemed ahead of time to be non-refundable. The other advantage of a retainer is that the payment is completely separated from the outcome of the analysis (Lubet 1998). As such, during testimony, the expert makes it clear that the payment could not have been as significantly influential over the determination as one where payment follows the opinion.

Some jurisdictions do not support the use of retainers in criminal cases, where they are seen as exploitative. The practice of retaining an expert can also be used to actively exclude experts from further participation in a case (Ainsworth 2010). Lawyers may seek to limit the range of experts available to the opposing side by "locking up" those that may be most influential to a case. This practice does raise access-to-justice concerns, which is outside the purview of this chapter.

In some cases, the expert is retained, and upon completion of their analysis renders an opinion that is inconsistent with the expectations of the party who retained them. As the expert's opinion does not support that party's theory of the case, the retaining party may simply discharge the expert, or make very limited (or none at all) further use of the expert's services. The expert is ethically precluded from consulting the opposing party, and therefore loses the opportunity for further compensation in the case. To protect against this occurrence, some experts demand a non-refundable fee, recognizing the financial risk they face if their participation is limited (Ainsworth 2010; Lubet 1998).

### 12.2.2   Fee for service

Fee for service charges can be calculated on a per hour or per case basis – to be agreed upon prior to accepting a case. The Forensic Anthropologist should have a clear understanding of the work being requested while the agency requesting service should have an idea of the overall cost and the timeframe involved. A contract or Fee Agreement is advisable (see the Appendix for an example of a Fee Agreement) and should be discussed, agreed upon and signed by both parties prior to the acceptance of a case.

Typical costs, usually calculated on an hourly basis, include the preparation, analysis, and documentation of a case, preparation of the case report, pretrial conferences, depositions, and preparation of presentations before the case actually reaches the courtroom (Matson 2012; Murphy 2000). At present, there are no agreed-upon or professionally endorsed fees for Forensic Anthropology services. The amount of the hourly fee for service varies depending on budget allowances, the experience level of the anthropologist, and the types of service provided (i.e. mass fatality response may demand a larger fee per hour than typical scene response). Typical hourly fees could range from $100 per hour for initial case analysis and review to $350 per hour for depositions, and $500 per hour for trial testimony.

Alternatively, fees can be set on the basis of the type of material to be examined or the duty to be performed by the expert (Table 12.1). In these cases, the flat fee is invoked whether the case actually takes less time or more time than anticipated. The benefit is that the client knows, in advance, the fees due. This

**Table 12.1** Example of fee schedule with a combination of hour or daily fees and flat fees.

| Type of service | Cost |
| --- | --- |
| Email/photograph consultation | $50–250 |
| Non-human, with case report | $100–500 |
| Full examination of complete skeletal remains (>50% complete) | $1000–5000 |
| Full examination of partial skeletal remains (<50% complete) | $750–2000 |
| Full examination of single postcranial bone | $200–500 |
| Skull only, non-forensic | $350–750 |
| Skull only, forensic | $450–1000 |
| Partial examination of skeletal remains | $500–1500 |
| Trauma evaluation of skeletal remains | $500–2000 |
| Radiographic examination/comparison | $350–1000 |
| Consultation at autopsy, no case report | $250–750 |
| Consultation at autopsy, with case report | $350–1000 |
| Scene response | $100–500 $h^{-1}$ |
| Mass fatality response | $200–500 $h^{-1}$ |
| Exhumation | $1500–3000 $d^{-1}$ |
| Pretrial conference | $200–500 $h^{-1}$ |
| Deposition | $200–500 $h^{-1}$ |
| Court testimony travel, wait, and preparation time | $75–200 $h^{-1}$ |
| Court testimony | $300–700+ $h^{-1}$ |
| Other analyses as requested | Variable |

Amounts will vary depending on a number of factors and will change over time.

may be helpful when there are budgets to be considered or when counsel must petition for approval of the use of an expert witness.

Trial costs would include the time on the stand, but also include waiting time in the courthouse, any last minute conferencing and transportation times. Some experts also charge on a "port-to-port" basis so expenses begin at an hourly rate from the time the expert leaves their home site until they return (Matson 2012).

Often a minimum time is charged. For example, a charge for two hours may be imposed even if the actual court time is relatively short. This minimum acknowledges the investment that the expert has devoted to the preparation and does not rush testimony. Usually the time actually spent is also rounded up although individuals may choose to do this on full hour, half hour, or quarter hour increments. Another option is to provide a daily rate regardless of the amount of time spent in court. Furthermore, charging a flat fee for trial, which includes travel time, may remediate any concerns about potential double billing when the expert may be working on multiple cases at one time.

For cases where the expert is being retained and paid through a government agency, there may be serious restrictions on the allowable hourly fees or the way that the fees are calculated. For example, some states impose a maximum hourly fee for testimony. These issues should be clarified prior to the agreement.

### 12.2.3 Fee for service considerations

One significant consideration when requiring fee for service is the interaction between that fee, the individual performing the analysis and the institution that is the regular employer of the individual. For many anthropologists, this institution is the college or university or the coroner/medical examiner's office for which they work. The first concern is the amount of outside work that can be provided. Many universities recognize that outside employment is a benefit to their faculty in more than financial terms. Such work keeps people current with their fields and provides real world examples for them to bring to the classroom. Understanding the limits on time or income, how impacts on normal employment responsibilities are being handled, and reporting structures for outside income should be investigated prior to accepting cases. Some institutions, such as universities, expect faculty experts to testify on their own time, ideally so there is no conflict with teaching schedules or service work.

Experts who work for a medical examiner or coroner's office may have to disclose their outside work and, in some cases, obtain approval prior to engaging in private consulting. There are two causes for concern here: one is the potential for a conflict of interest and the other is that, for certain disciplines, such as forensic pathology for instance, the outside work counts as part of the overall caseload of the physician and the combination of outside casework and regular duty casework may exceed the allowed maximums for accreditation by the

National Association of Medical Examiners. In the first case, experts employed by a medical examiner/coroner are typically not permitted to consult on any criminal case that was investigated by their office, even if they had no prior involvement. Similarly, any civil litigation that might arise from a case investigated by their employer is considered off limits due to conflict of interest. Regardless of the party approaching an expert for expert advice, any potential for conflict of interest or ethical irregularities should be considered prior to accepting the case.

Distinction must also be made as to where and with what equipment the anthropologist is working. If the anthropologist is utilizing the resources of their home institution, the institution is entitled to some compensation. Some agencies will allow such work on a very limited basis but as it becomes more significant, there should be cost sharing whereby a portion of the income is returned to the institution. However, if equipment was purchased by the expert with their own money, they could conduct casework off campus at the location requesting their services, and be compensated accordingly.

Similarly, when working for one government agency, equipment, and/or lab space belonging to that agency may not be used to conduct analysis for another government agency or for a private entity whose case does not fall under the jurisdiction of the employer. For example, if a Forensic Anthropologist is asked to conduct a cremains analysis outside of their employment to determine if commingling occurred they may not use their employer's laboratory, work-space computer, or any equipment to perform the examination.

When working as a paid outside consultant, the use of vacation time or personal time is also a factor. Institutions, especially those that are tax-payer funded, often frown on deriving income from two sources for the same time period unless specifically allowed. For academic positions, which normally do not accrue vacation time, permission to work away from normal duties is required. It is advisable to understand the restrictions on paid and unpaid time away from the home agency or institution and acceptance of outside consultations prior to embarking on such work.

When forensic anthropological casework is a large component of the anthropologist's time and responsibilities within an institution, it is customary for the fees from outside sources to be paid to the institution. Agreements with institutional administrations may allow for these funds, or large portions of them, to be returned to the laboratory for supplies, personal protective equipment, equipment upgrades, professional development, student training, and other expenses that may be beyond the means of the institution to provide. Such arrangements are beneficial to both the institution and the anthropologist but must be arranged before accepting casework.

How to set the scale of the fees is often a difficult subject as fees range widely between expert witnesses (Shuman et al. 1994). Some are clearly exorbitant

(Richmond 1999). In some cases, the courts have looked at the equivalent annual salary based on an hourly rate to determine whether the "salary" is multiples of a normal annual income of a professional in that field.

On the flip side, very low fees may allow the attorneys to waste the time of the expert by extending time on the stand, pretrial conferences, or in depositions (Matson 2012; Richmond 1999). For example, if waiting time is charged at a very low rate, the anthropologist may well be kept on hold while more important (i.e. "more expensive") witnesses are given priority. Courts will support a minimum that is sufficiently significant that attorneys do not draw out questioning or waiting unreasonably.

When looking for comparisons of fees charged among expert witnesses, the Forensic Anthropologist should bear in mind differences between criminal and civil cases, the latter often investing more in hopes of later financial return. As stated elsewhere, some states have set amounts that they are willing to pay for services and fee structures will reflect the permissible scale in the area in which the expert usually works. Fee scales in civil cases tend to look at a number of factors in determining the amount available for service including area of expertise, education, prevailing rates, complexity of the work, and whether the expert charges different fees for different agencies (Richmond 1999).

Despite widespread belief that scientific expert witnesses customarily charge extremely high fees and derive much of their income from such fees, in most cases, the fees are far short of exorbitant levels and few experts make the majority of their income from expert testimony (Champagne et al. 1992). For the majority of experts in the courts, this source is a relatively small commitment in both income and time invested compared with their normal duties.

When the expert testifies but has not received payment for the analysis upon which the testimony is based, there may be the impression that the expert may want to ensure payment by testifying in a manner that is acceptable or preferable to the side soliciting the service (Preber 2014). As we will discuss in Section 12.4, one should consider that all bills be paid prior to testimony. This will reduce any appearance of impropriety.

### 12.2.4   Pro bono

For many people working intermittently in forensic case work but whose primary employment is not directly tied to the forensic sciences, one option may be to avoid charging for the bulk of their services. The decision to do so will depend on the source of funding, the complexity of handling income from outside the primary place of employment and alternative ways to value the services provided within the recognition systems of the home agency.

In these cases, use of institutional facilities and equipment for forensic work is usually acceptable as it is seen as part of the requirement of employees to participate in public service. The downside of this approach is that there is usually little commitment on the part of the institution to invest further in the facilities even when they are delighted to highlight the work in promotional material.

The "pro bono" approach can be combined with some fee-charging activities by not charging for the analysis of material and production of the case report but making an expectation for some compensation for court testimony and associated duties along with expenses. During these times, the expert would need to be on leave or use vacation time from the institution for the duration of their court work and must file appropriate paperwork recognizing outside income. In addition to these options, some experts may charge for some services, such as the skeletal analysis and report writing, but not for others (e.g. processing time, search, and recovery). Discounting the fee schedule is a further option, especially for jurisdictions that have small budgets for forensic services. This may be justifiable for laboratories that rely in large part on student or intern labor to assist with tasks such as processing remains and photography.

One consideration, if this avenue is explored, is that other Forensic Anthropologists who do not work for an academic institution or government agency will be asked for comparison figures when submitting their fee schedule. Practitioners who do not charge for their expertise may undermine the ability of others to earn a reasonable wage. To accommodate these factors, one recommendation would be to submit an invoice listing the fees for service and then zeroing out the invoice. This practice demonstrates the value of the work without actual cost to the requesting party.

### 12.2.5    Reasonable expenses

Normal expenses should be provided to the expert witness for both analysis and testimony, and should be consistent from agency to agency. Some experts charge a nominal supplies fee to agencies, even when not charging for services, in order to cover the cost of expendable items such as gloves, personal protective equipment, plastic sheeting, and soft tissue disposal along with utilities for the laboratory. For scene response and court testimony where travel is involved, additional expenses should be anticipated, including travel and hotel. In many circumstances, the expert purchases the items needed (e.g. airline tickets, rental cars, hotel, parking, taxi/ride-sharing expenses) and bills the agency for these costs. Some government agencies have separate arrangements with travel providers and will purchase tickets for the expert and may also book them into hotels. Government agencies may also have restrictions on the level of transportation provided, such as economy class airfares or compact rental cars.

The cost of food should also be considered. A per diem cost for overnight or out of state travel is often expected to cover hotel and food expenses. This rate can be based on standard published government per diem amounts. Alternatively, the expert may need to submit specific receipts of food purchased.

Additional expenses outside those incurred for the testimony cannot be billed to the agency. Extending a stay beyond that needed for court, deposition or analysis is acceptable in order to enjoy the location but charging the additional amounts to the agency are not. Time sheets should be maintained and submitted with the invoice to account for all of the charged fees.

In most cases, additional expenses such as childcare or pet sitting are not allowed. In many cases, alcohol cannot be paid for by state funds, so drinks purchased during the course of the case work are not allowable. Similarly, entertainment costs are not allowable if not directly related to the case. Upgrades in hotel rooms, airline tickets, and rental cars may be the responsibility of the expert rather than the funding agency unless there are specific reasons for the changes and these are agreed to prior to travel. If the expert is traveling to a rural area with no easy means of getting to the hotel or the courthouse, the agency should be tasked with providing transportation.

## 12.3  Unethical billing practices

There are three compensation practices that are generally seen as unethical or, at least, inadvisable. The first is the use of "contingency fees," meaning that fees are dependent on the outcome of the case (Ainsworth 2010; Lubet 1998; Parker 1990). This fee structure provides an incentive for the expert to tailor their opinion to meet the preferred argument to the side for whom they are presenting, in order to get any payment. A variant on this unacceptable approach is when fees are rebated if the expert's opinion rendered is not considered appropriate for the case as seen by the employing attorneys. The American Bar Association's Model Code further states that it is improper for experts to work on a contingency basis (Murphy 2000).

The second area of questionable practice is "value billing" (Lubet 1998). In value billing, the fees are determined by the value of the testimony to the side employing the expert, again, providing an incentive to tailor testimony to increase the value of the opinion to the attorneys. Forensic Anthropologists should be aware of these unethical approaches and should not agree to these fees. Forensic Anthropologists also should be aware that the manner in which they are compensated is admissible at trial, and the use of either contingency fees or value billing generates an immediate (and effective) circumstance by which the expert's credibility may be attacked. And this assumes that an opinion developed by the expert being compensated in this manner would survive a challenge under *Daubert* or *Frye*.

A third highly questionable area is double billing for time or expenses. For example, time waiting outside the courtroom for one case may be spent working on another but double billing both cases for the same time is unethical. Expenses can also fall into the realm of double billing (Gutheil et al. 1998). The expert may be flying to one location, traveling on to another and then returning from the second location to their home base. The question is how to allocate the cost of the various legs of the flight appropriately without double billing. Potential options should be discussed with the clients before expenses are incurred and invoices sent.

## 12.4   Invoicing

One of the most challenging aspects of setting up a consulting practice is figuring out how to get paid. Forensic Anthropologists working outside of an academic institution or medical examiner/coroner office are confronted with the fact that they have to develop a workable billing system for their services. Important considerations include setting up a fee schedule, time tracking while working on a case or cases, determining how often to submit invoices, ensuring that they are paid in a timely fashion and deciding on a mechanism for payment. As consultants, practitioners may also be asked to provide proof of insurance and workers compensation, but this varies by state. Typically, because the Forensic Anthropologist does not have any employees and insurance costs more than any profit earned from the work, waivers can be signed for both insurance and workers compensation. However, some agencies still require sizable insurance packages before retaining an anthropologist as a regular consultant.

A fee agreement lays out the responsibilities of each party bound by the contract. Usually it includes the names of the parties, a description of the work to be performed, expenses that are to be included, a fee schedule, the timelines for the work to be completed, a billing address, a schedule for invoicing and the penalty amount for late payments (see Appendix).

Organization is key when developing your billing system. Checklists or spreadsheets are an easy way to track each case and can be attached to the file digitally or in paper form. The fee agreement should be signed by both parties, and can be notarized for extra protection, prior to any exchange of documents or case material for analysis and/or review. The Forensic Anthropologist should have an easy way to track the time spent on the case and it should be divided into the type of activity. For example, review of the case material might be billed at a different rate than time spent on the phone with the attorney. Research or literature review might be less expensive than case file review or physical analysis. Travel might be billed at a lower rate than waiting or actual time spent testifying. All of those areas must be documented and reflected on the invoice.

Often cases wend through the court system very slowly so invoicing can be done incrementally rather than all together at the conclusion of the expert's involvement. The overall length of the review (days, weeks, months, years) will dictate the schedule for sending an invoice. Typically, an invoice would be sent once a month, but if the analysis only requires two days, the invoice can be sent immediately. As mentioned elsewhere in the chapter, all analytical work performed before the date of trial should be invoiced and paid prior to the actual courtroom testimony. The time needed to prepare for trial, including pretrial meetings and phone calls, are typically billed along with the fees and expenses for the testimony itself.

Payment can be requested "upon receipt" or by a certain date after submission. The expert should have a mechanism to track payments which can be tendered by cash, check, credit card, direct deposit, or through an online payment system. A receipt should be provided by the expert. The tracking system should include some type of notification if a payment is late. Attorneys are notoriously tardy with payment so the expert will have to regularly monitor all outstanding invoices. A late fee can be charged if it is included in the original fee agreement.

## 12.5   The professional expert

Traditionally, in Forensic Anthropology, expert testimony is requested by the prosecutor in a criminal trial because the findings bolster their theory of the case. In more recent times, there are increasing demands for forensic science services; partly to provide even access to justice and partly because more members of the defense bar recognize experts as important to their case. In response, many forensic scientists have established independent laboratories that primarily service the defense community although they are available to all interested parties. This professional expert is often confronted with questions regarding their source of income that may be entirely derived from casework and/or predominately for one "side" or the other. As with all such matters, the professional expert should be forthright about their fee structure and clear that they are being recompensed for their time, not their opinion. Courts have allowed some questioning about overall income, income from specific cases, and income from specific law practices so the expert should be prepared. Full disclosure of personal finances is problematic as they expose the expert to subsequent abuse (Richmond 1999). Pursuit of such lines of questioning are often seen as attempts to intimidate the witness and courts may restrict the scope of such questioning.

Every discipline within the forensic sciences has concerns about those who may appear or who may actually be willing to provide testimony solely per the request of either prosecution or defense. While this may play out in terms of ethics, it also makes an appearance in the guise of fees. Experts who provide competent, non-biased reviews, and rely on their professional consultations for income are often painted with the same brush as those who are willing to sell a favorable opinion to the highest bidder. One of the responsibilities of the hiring attorney is to bring this distinction out during the direct examination.

Thus, two questions are brought to the fore: (i) how does an expert witness protect against a claim that an opinion has been bought; and (ii) how can attorneys recognize the need to question those who may be willing to skew their findings to the side of the highest bidder. The indication that potentially unethical behavior has occurred is not in how fees are charged but rather when the fees are combined with dubious methodology or interpretation, inappropriate conclusions, or practices that are clearly not the norm within the discipline (Richmond 1999). Many Forensic Anthropologists are reluctant to value their time appropriately for fear that they will be seen as providing an opinion for the money. The secret to the ethical stance, however, does not lie in charging reasonable fees for service but in the professional and ethical practice of the discipline. Attorneys usually will not work for free and it is not reasonable for experts to do so either. Matter of fact presentation of a fee agreement along with a clearly stated fee structure precludes any misunderstandings. Placing a reasonable monetary value on time spent and knowledge shared both helps to change the perception of the attorneys and the jury regarding the testimony and helps to prepare the expert for disparaging cross-examination. Understanding the difference between charging for time spent and knowledge shared and charging for a favorable opinion can also assist the expert in preparing counsel to cross-examine the opposing expert.

## 12.6  Conclusions

The Forensic Anthropologist provides a valuable service for the legal community by analyzing skeletal material, providing information regarding the biological profile, documenting evidence of traumatic injury to the decedent, providing a reliable estimation of the time since death and other events that might have happened to the body following death. As with all experts, the individual practitioner should be compensated for their time but not for their opinion. By creating and regularly updating a fee schedule for different types of analyses or work product and providing an up-front fee agreement that clearly outlines the expectations for each party, the expert can avoid many of the pitfalls that come from providing testimony. Forensic Anthropologists should value their time and expertise and expect compensation for the work they have done in the analysis and interpretation of evidence.

## 12.A  Appendix

An example of a fee agreement

Date: _____ Name of attorney(s) _____

Case #/ Name_____

Office name/address:_____

Telephone #: _____     Fax #: _____

I understand that Dr. _____ charges for time spent in both preparation for and participation in expert consultation and/or legal proceedings. This includes any activity relating to legal actions in these matters, and includes interviews with myself or another representative of my law firm (in person or via long-distance communications), depositions with same (at subpoena of myself or my firm), court proceedings, and time spent preparing for the above.

I further understand that cancellation or postponement of previously scheduled interviews, conferences, depositions, or court testimony without sufficient prior notice may still incur charges if Dr. _____ has spent time preparing for the above, and if travel or other related expenses have already been paid by Dr. _____ in anticipation of such proceedings. The charges for these services are as follows:

$ _____ per hour or portion thereof for preparation/consultation conferences/communications

$ _____ minimum for first two hours of deposition or trial testimony;

$ _____ for each additional hour or portion thereof of testimony

$ _____ minimum per day*, plus standard travel expenses** as incurred when traveling for meetings or testimony, with actual testimony time reimbursed as above

*       Includes waiting time and time spent in travel, when incurred, as a result of consultation and/or preparation for, or actual participation in deposition or court proceedings; assumes an 8 hour working day; extra time involved on case-related issues will incur additional billing.

**       Includes standard airfare, rental or personal car expenses, food, and lodging when necessary.

I also understand that late fees (10 % of base fee per month overdue) and all collections costs will be paid by my firm, if applicable.

Signature: _____ Date: _____

Please Make Check Payable to: _____

# References

Ainsworth, J. (2010). A lawyer's perspective: ethical, technical, and practical considerations in the use of linguistic expert witnesses. *International Journal of Speech Language and the Law* 16 (2): 279–291.

Champagne, A., Shuman, D., and Whitaker, E. (1992). Expert witnesses in the courts: an empirical examination. *Judicature* 76 (1): 5–10.

Golan, T. (1999). The history of scientific expert testimony in the English courtroom. *Science in Context* I (1): 7–32.

Golan, T. (2008). Revisiting the history of scientific expert testimony. *Brooklyn Law Review* 73 (3): 879–942.

Graham, M.H. (1977). Impeaching the professional expert witness by a showing of financial interest. *Indiana Law Journal* 53 (1): 35–53.

Gutheil, T.G., Slater, F.E., Commons, M.L., and Goodheart, E.A. (1998). Expert witness travel dilemmas: a pilot study of billing practices. *Journal of the American Academy of Psychiatry and the Law* 26 (1): 21–26.

Lubet, S. (1998). Expert witnesses: ethics and professionalism. *Georgetown Law Review* 12 (3): 465–488.

Matson, J.V. (2012). *Effective Expert Witnessing: Practices for the 21st Century*. Boca Raton, FL: CRC Press.

Morgan, W.G. (1953). Expert witness fees. *The Journal of Criminal Law, Criminology, and Police Science* 43 (6): 777–783.

Murphy, J.P. (2000). Expert witnesses at trial: where are the ethics? *Georgetown Journal of Legal Ethics* 14: 217–239.

Parker, J.J. (1990). Contingent expert witness fees: access and legitimacy. *Southern California Law Review* 64: 1363–1391.

Preber, B.J. (2014). *Financial Expert Witness Communication: a Practical Guide to Reporting and Testimony*. Hoboken, NJ: Wiley.

Richmond, D.R. (1999). Expert witness conflicts and compensation. *Tennessee Law Review* 67: 909–948.

Shuman, D.W., Whitaker, E., and Champagne, A. (1994). An empirical examination of the use of expert witnesses in the courts – Part II: a three city study. *Jurimetrics Journal* 34 (2): 193–208.

# Index

---

*Forensic Anthropology and the United States Judicial System*, First Edition.
Edited by Laura C. Fulginiti, Kristen Hartnett-McCann, and Alison Galloway.
© 2019 John Wiley & Sons Ltd. Published 2019 by John Wiley & Sons Ltd.